An Overview of Early Intervention

An Overview of Early Intervention

E.J. Brown

with Jane Sorensen, PhD, OTR, ND

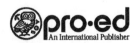
pro·ed
An International Publisher

8700 Shoal Creek Boulevard
Austin, Texas 78757-6897
800/897-3202   Fax 800/397-7633
www.proedinc.com

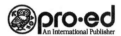

© 2007 by PRO-ED, Inc.
8700 Shoal Creek Boulevard
Austin, Texas 78757-6897
800/897-3202   Fax 800/397-7633
www.proedinc.com

The authors gratefully acknowledge permission to reprint the following
copyrighted material:
NECTAC List of Part C Lead Agencies © 2005 by National Early Childhood
    Technical Assistance Center.
She Loves Me, She Loves Me Not . . . © 2002 by *ADVANCE for
    Occupational Therapy Practitioners,* Merion Publications, Inc.
On the Sidelines © 2001 by *ADVANCE for Occupational Therapy
    Practitioners,* Merion Publications, Inc.
Of A Different Mind © 2003 by *ADVANCE for Occupational Therapy
    Practitioners,* Merion Publications, Inc.
Welcome to Holland © 1987 Emily Perl Kingsley.
The 12 Theories of Learning © Funderstanding.
Zero to Three © Mark L. Batshaw

Library of Congress Cataloging-in-Publication Data

Brown, E. J.
    An overview of early intervention / E.J. Brown with Jane Sorensen.
        p. ; cm.
        Includes bibliographical references.
        ISBN-13: 978-1-4164-0334-0
        ISBN-10: 1-4164-0334-5
    1. Occupational therapy for children.   2. Infants with disabilities.
    I. Sorensen, Jane. II. Title.
    [DNLM: 1. Early Intervention (Education)   2. Occupational Therapy.
    3. Child, Preschool.   4. Infant. WS 368 B877o 2007]
    RJ53.O25B76 2007
    649'.6—dc22
                                    2006031393

Printed in the United States of America

1 2 3 4 5 6 7 8 9 10   10 09 08 07 06

Table of Contents

Introduction

This book is an overview of home-based early intervention (EI) in occupational therapy for children 0–3 years old. You may choose to read this book for many reasons. Perhaps you are a student seeking to learn the basics of working with the 0–3 population, an experienced practitioner who desires to change practice settings, or an educator who would like to include this field in your coursework. Whatever the case, we hope you will find what you are looking for and more in this book.

Occupational therapists (OT) and therapy assistants can use this book as a formal educational tool in the classroom or for self-study. Each chapter includes questions meant to be used as a springboard for discussion or further investigation. We hope that those of you who have chosen this practice for your first job in the OT profession, or who feel somewhat isolated from your colleagues working in EI, will gain a new perspective of your job from reading this book, and with it, a greater confidence in your skills. But what we really hope to do is inspire you and allow you to see and feel how much you are needed in this particular treatment arena.

The basic goals for the EI work setting have already been set in place for you in the Individuals with Disabilities Education Act (IDEA), which the U.S. Congress has recently reauthorized, but how you use the law is really up to you. This book will give you an overview of the act and how it empowers you to help the families of infants and toddlers referred to you for evaluation or treatment. Here are some of the things we hope you will learn:

- In home-based early intervention you are first and foremost a teacher. It is your job to evaluate child development patterns in the families you see, and then to teach parents how to participate with their children in the therapeutic activities. This will help those children reach their fullest potential in the earliest years of life.

- You will discover how to listen to parents and find out what kind of help they are seeking for their child and what they hope to achieve. In each home you will learn what to look for to evaluate family functioning patterns and how to offer parents, through your own skills or referral to other specialists, the help they need to achieve a satisfying and nurturing relationship with their child. This is, in fact, one of the basic goals of IDEA.

- Early intervention is not meant to overburden families with so much help that they no longer have control of their lives. All home-based care works best when specialists function as a team, not just a group, to provide targeted help to families. This is necessary not only to provide the best care, but to keep the costs of that care at a reasonable level. You, as a therapist or therapy assistant, can help your team, or the agency for which you work, learn to use this team model.

In this book you will soon discover why "people skills" are the most important ones you will use as you interact with the children you see, their parents, your colleagues, and your employers.

Home-based early intervention can be one of the most satisfying job arenas for you as a therapist because you are working in natural environments where parents and children actually do their living—their homes, on their streets, in their parks, and wherever they regularly interact with one another. To be effective, however, you will find that you need to be proactive in communicating with others working on your cases, and that you need to be flexible in recognizing and adapting to changing family circumstances and priorities.

Good luck in your career, and if you have not already done so, we hope we will inspire you will try early intervention as a practice setting.

E. J. Brown

Jane Sorensen, PhD, OTR, ND

Understanding Early Intervention, Achieving Best Practice

1

SUSAN'S STORY

Susan was speaking with an older mother whose 6-week-old baby had severe birth defects. An amniocentesis during the mother's seventh month of pregnancy had revealed chromosomal abnormalities. In addition to these abnormalities, the little girl had been born with hydrocephalus, was not able to feed from a bottle, and had had a feeding tube inserted directly into her stomach. By all indicators, the child's prognosis was not good.

Susan, an experienced occupational therapist (OT), had just begun working in early intervention (EI) and had not encountered many of these children in her career. Although only a few years ago these infants would not have survived, advances in medical care had saved this child's life. However, she would have profound mental retardation. Though the neonatologist had informed the mother of this while the baby was in the neo-natal intensive care unit (NICU), Mom still found it difficult to fully comprehend the situation.

Susan was not there to force the mother to accept the infant's prognosis. Rather, she needed to teach the mother how to stimulate visual tracking as outlined in the baby's individualized family service plan (IFSP). When Susan began to discuss the baby's therapy, the mother interrupted, asking, "I really want my little girl to have as normal a life as possible. Do you think she'll be able to have children when she grows up?"

Susan now faced a dilemma common to EI therapists and other service providers. No matter what she answered, it would be wrong. She looked at the woman, her clinical reasoning took over, and she fell back on some insightful humor. "My goodness," she said, "she isn't even menstruating!"

The mother laughed, and the immediate crisis was over. They went back to talking about visual tracking issues, and Susan was thankful for her training in psychology. Such moments are common in EI. The role of an EI therapist is not only to help children from birth to age three get a good start educationally, but also to help their families learn to take over that task. Sometimes helping a family means more than following the treatment goals set forth in an IFSP.

Therapists working in early intervention (EI) use all of their skills every day. In the case above, Susan's training in psychology enabled her to evaluate the mother's state of mind quickly and accurately. "This mom was too fragile for a 'your child will need lifelong care' talk," Susan said. "But if I had gone along with her, it would have reinforced her denial. Denial is normal this early in the game, so I answered with a little humorous reality and did not give false hope."

Inexperienced therapists can be overwhelmed by having to respond appropriately, professionally, and compassionately in an emotionally-wrought situation. Instead of engaging with parents like the mother above, these therapists might fall back on what makes them comfortable and refuse to discuss anything outside the written outcomes they are there to help the child achieve. When EI therapists define the boundaries of their work so strictly, practice becomes rote, and they miss numerous opportunities to help the family heal and grow together.

Is Early Intervention Right for You?

Perhaps the most important characteristic of people who work successfully in early intervention is independence. Much of EI is home-based therapy, and there are big differences between the home environment and the clinic. For occupational therapists, physical therapists, and speech-language pathologists, EI is similar to home care in some respects; however, EI is based on an educational model that is meant to be more preventive than curative. Unlike school-based therapy, EI does not work around a team, even though a team is involved in the evaluation and intervention. Because EI therapists work independently, anyone considering switching to this field or re-entering the profession in this arena should find a mentor. Ideally, you should arrange to accompany an EI therapist on rounds to get a feel for the practice setting before going out alone.

Successful therapists are the ones who know their fields well enough to lead their client's families and to educate agency personnel in best-practice principles and protocols, if necessary. Although many agencies try to provide some kind of mentoring program for their therapists, there are usually no supervisors or administrators present to tell therapists how to practice their trade, as is the case with hospital personnel. Instead, EI therapists use their best clinical judgments, make the best case for their choices, and convince case managers and agency personnel of their expertise. A successful EI therapist must be highly interested in and committed to his or her job.

"Best practice" in early intervention means a commitment to an overarching approach to evaluation and treatment that follows the spirit of Part C of the *Individuals With Disabilities Education Act* (IDEA), 1986. This is the federal law that supports assessment and treatment of children from birth to 3 years (36 months) old to help parents and caregivers learn to care appropriately for their children who are disabled or developmentally delayed, and to relate well to those children. Treatment is usually performed in the home Best practice also means promoting a true team approach to care. If your employer does not have a team-based system in place, open a dialogue on a case-by-case basis with necessary partners in treatment—agency personnel, other disciplines, family members, equipment providers, physicians and/or case managers—to clarify goals, troubleshoot, or streamline services when necessary.

Understanding IDEA

Congress first passed IDEA in 1975, thereby assuring children with disabilities the right to a free public education equal to that of their non-disabled peers. The 0–3 population has only been covered since 1986, when Congress amended the act to include what is now Part C, Infants and Toddlers with Disabilities. Up to that time, preschool therapy had been considered "early intervention," but the costs of educating children with disabilities were increasing annually. Educators hoped to reduce these costs by correcting some problems early on so that these children might enter the classroom with the greatest degree of functional mobility and cognition. Today, IDEA is the foundation of all early intervention programs, and it is essential for practitioners in the field to understand its mandates.

How IDEA Is Administered

Lawmakers set up a somewhat complicated structure for the administration of early intervention because children in this age group spend most of their time at home: The family unit is their school; their parents and other caregivers are their teachers. As a "related service" in the educational setting, therapy has had to concentrate on educational goals rather than health goals, but the dividing line between physical development and educational readiness is almost nonexistent in early intervention. Under the act, states are free to assign responsibility for IDEA Part C to agencies other than their departments of education. In 36 states Part C is administered by health, welfare, rehabilitation, and other departments (National Early Childhood Technical Assistance Center, 2003).

The Mandate for Family-Centered Care

Though infants and toddlers may be treated in centralized settings, Part C makes it clear that the environment is to be kept as "natural" as possible. Basically, that means the environment should be the home. Here, the parents, not the doctors or the therapists, rule.

> The contents of the individualized family service plan shall be fully explained to the parents, and informed written consent from the parents shall be obtained prior to the provision of early intervention services described in such plan. If the parents do not provide consent with respect to a particular early intervention service, then the early intervention services to which consent is obtained shall be provided. (Public Law 105–17, Sec. 636e)

The outcomes sought in early intervention are determined by the wishes of the parents. Their goals may not always seem realistic to medically trained personnel, but the parents' goals are what the therapists should aim to achieve. No matter what is indicated in the IFSP, the parents may choose to ignore any part they disagree with or dislike.

Parents ultimately determine the course of their child's therapy, and EI therapists must be prepared to work not only with children with disabilities, but also with their families. IDEA clearly encourages not only the evaluation of children referred to the program, but of their families as well. Under Section 636 of IDEA, the statewide system set up to administer the law states that state agencies, at a minimum, should provide a family-directed assessment of resources, priorities and concerns of the family, and the identification of the supports and services necessary to enhance family's capacity to meet the developmental needs of the infant or toddler. Family evaluation is voluntary (as is the whole program), and unless the state has spent time and effort in initiating this part of the program, most families opt out of it. This may be due to the parents' fear the evaluation will somehow find them lacking, as though they will be held responsible for precipitating or reinforcing their child's problem.

What's New in the Law

Individuals With Disabilities Education Improvement Act (PL 108–446), the latest reauthorization of IDEA, became law on December 3, 2004. Part C has seen some subtle, but significant changes. Congress found a substantial need to recognize the significant brain development that occurs during a child's first few years of life, and to note that all children are now covered by IDEA, rather than just "historically underrepresented populations;" homeless and foster-care children are now specifically identified. Early intervention services are to be established based on scientific research, to the extent practicable. The American Occupational Therapy Association (AOTA) and other EI therapy disciplines helped add the wording "to the extent practicable" so that interventions that are not proven to the highest medical standards would be allowed.

Some parents whose children were in preschool programs such as Head Start can now choose home-based services for their children instead. Children may now remain in EI, with the written consent of parents, until they enter kindergarten. Personnel in EI are to be trained to coordinate transition services to preschool after age 3. States are free to enact guidelines that allow them to keep children in EI until they reach elementary school. Additionally, hospitals and physicians must make information on EI available to the parents of children with disabilities. The law also makes changes in funding mechanisms. Information about and a comparison of IDEA 1997 and the 2004 reauthorization is available from the US Department of Education (www.ed.gov/policy/speced/guid/idea/ides2004.html).

IDEA at a Glance

Goals of Early Intervention for Infants and Toddlers

1. Enhance development of infants and toddlers with disabilities and minimize their potential for developmental delay.

2. Reduce educational costs by minimizing the need for special education and related services once children reach school age.

3. Minimize the likelihood of institutionalization of individuals with disabilities.

4. Enhance the capacity of families to meet the special needs of their infants and toddlers with disabilities.

5. Enhance the ability of state and local agencies and service providers to identify, evaluate, and meet the needs of historically underrepresented populations (i.e., minority, low-income, inner-city, and rural populations).

The Department of Education's Role In Early Intervention

The U.S. Department of Education provides financial assistance to the states to:

- develop and implement a statewide, comprehensive, coordinated, multidisciplinary interagency system that provides EI services for infants and toddlers and their families,

- facilitate the coordination of payment for EI services from federal, state, local, and private sources (including public and private insurance coverage),

- enhance the states' capacity to provide quality EI services and expand and improve existing services being provided to infants and toddlers with disabilities and their families,

- encourage the states to expand opportunities for children under age 3 who would be at risk of having substantial developmental delay if they did not receive EI services.

Determining Eligibility for Early Intervention Services and How the Law Defines Services

Children from birth to age 3 who have, or are at risk for, developmental delays are eligible for government-subsidized EI services. An "at-risk infant or toddler" refers to a child 3 years old or younger who "would be at risk of experiencing a substantial developmental delay if early intervention services were not provided to the individual" (IDEA, 2004, Sec. 632). The definition of "developmental delay," however, is left up to the states. The delay, as determined by testing, must be more than a certain percentage or must deviate from a mean standard of skill by a certain number. Children with a 33% delay or more in one developmental area, or with at least a 25% delay in two or more areas, are usually eligible for EI services. "Early intervention services means developmental services," according to Section 632 of IDEA. These services must be provided under public supervision, at no cost (unless the state initiates a sliding fee scale), and can address development in five categories: physical, cognitive, communicative, social/emotional, and adaptive.

Under Section 641, IDEA requires governors to appoint lead agencies to receive grants and administer the program. States must also establish state interagency coordinating councils for the purpose of becoming eligible to receive funding. Governors appoint the council members, who represent the state's population in terms of sex and ethnicity reasonably well. The governors may appoint the council chairs or allow the councils to select their own chairs. Any member of the council who is a representative of the lead agency may not serve as chair.

How Part C, 0 to 3 Intervention, Is Similar to Early Intervention for 3- to 5-Year-Olds

Early intervention for children ages birth to 3 years old is meant to prepare children with physical and cognitive delays for school, but Part C is more family-centered. In fact, it gives the family almost total control over the process. The real intent of Part C is to show parents how to do the things that benefit their children's development the most. Its foundation lies in teaching parents child-handling skills and in therapeutic use of self to meet the psychosocial challenges that may keep these parents from performing their role successfully.

Who Can Provide Services

Pediatricians and other physicians, speech-language pathologists, occupational therapists, psychologists, social workers, nurses, nutritionists, family therapists, orientation and mobility specialists, service coordinators, and medical personnel (for diagnosis and evaluation) are named in the act as qualified providers. Children with delays are eligible for family training, counseling and home visits, special instruction, speech-language pathology and audiology, occupational therapy, physical therapy, psychological therapy, service coordination, social services, nursing, nutritional intervention, vision services, and transportation that enables families to gain access to these services. The state interagency coordinating council includes a personnel development member whose job it is to set educational standards. In the case of licensed personnel, those standards are already set.

How Early Intervention Providers Are Contracted and Paid

The lead agency, as designated by the governor of a state, is responsible for handing out funds. Therefore, the lead agency may make formal payment agreements with other eligible agencies to provide services in their areas.

Contracting Directly With the State

EI therapists may contract directly with the state. Under the law, state lead agencies are required to adopt policies that allow "other arrangements" with service providers, who nevertheless have to satisfy the requirements of Part C and those that are set forth in the application itself. Some local units reduce this option with administrative policies because private contractors cost more time and money to manage than agencies.

Where Early Intervention Services Are Provided and How Service Plans Are Developed

"To the maximum extent available," EI services are to take place in "natural environments," such as the home or "community settings in which children without disabilities participate," and they must be provided in accordance with the goals set by the children's IFSPs (IDEA, 2004, Sec. 635).

IFSPs differ from Individualized Education Programs (IEPs), with which school-based therapists work, in the following ways:

- Children may be evaluated for Part C solely at their parents' request.

- Families, not educators or therapists, direct the intervention by outlining their major concerns about their child and the outcomes they would like to see for that child (e.g., "I want to see him reach developmental milestones"). These parent-selected outcomes become the evaluating therapists' priorities in goal-setting. In fact, families may delete the goals they are not concerned about, even if evaluators have suggested they are necessary.

- Part C specifies that the IFSP should be "developed by a multidisciplinary team" but does not require the team to be physically together to do the job.

- A nurse, case manager, or other administrator of the agency through which a particular child is channeled for services, generally writes the plan. The IFSP does call for a "multidisciplinary assessment." In meetings with parents or other family members, agency administrators determine which disciplines they need to call on for evaluation, and then request such providers do written assessments. From these reports, the administrator and the family create the IFSP goals.

This means that unless you happen to be the administrator of an agency, you get no front-line observation under Part C. Someone else decides whether an evaluation from an early interventionist is necessary based on what he or she knows about your discipline. A definition of services is contained in section 303.12 of IDEA.

How the Lead Agency Differs From Other Participating Agencies

The lead agency is designated or established by the governor of a state to oversee the preparation and implementation of Part C, and to make sure that the state complies with IDEA standards. This body is responsible for supervising *all* Part C programming, whether or not the participants are claiming monies available for that purpose. That means identifying and coordinating all available resources within the state from federal, state, local, and private sources available for 0–3 intervention. The lead agency is usually a major department of the state, such as the health or education department (see Table 1.1 for the National Early Childhood Technical Assistance Center's [NECTAC] List of Lead Agencies).

Table 1.1 Early Intervention Lead Agencies by State

State/Jurisdiction	Lead Agency	State/Jurisdiction	Lead Agency
Alabama	Rehabilitation Services	Mississippi	Health
Alaska	Health and Social Services	Missouri	Education
American Samoa	Health	Montana	Public Health and Human Services
Arizona	Economic Security	Nebraska	Education and Health and Human Services (Co-Lead)
Arkansas	Human Services/Developmental Disabilities	Nevada	Human Resources/Health
California	Developmental Services	New Hampshire	Health and Human Services
Colorado	Education	New Jersey	Health and Senior Services
Commonwealth of Northern Mariana Islands	Education	New Mexico	Health
		New York	Health
Connecticut	Mental Retardation	North Carolina	Health and Human Services
Delaware	Health and Social Services	North Dakota	Human Services
District of Columbia	Human Services	Ohio	Health
Florida	Health (Children's Medical Services)	Oklahoma	Education
		Oregon	Education
Georgia	Human Resources/Division of Public Health	Pennsylvania	Public Welfare
		Puerto Rico	Health
Guam	Education	Rhode Island	Human Services
Hawaii	Health	South Carolina	Health and Environmental Control
Idaho	Health and Welfare/Developmental Disabilities	South Dakota	Education
		Tennessee	Education
Illinois	Human Services	Texas	Assistive and Rehabilitative Services
Indiana	Family and Social Services	Utah	Health
Iowa	Education	Vermont	Education and Human Services (Co-Lead)
Kansas	Health and Environment		
Kentucky	Health Services	Virgin Islands	Health
Louisiana	Health and Hospitals	Virginia	Mental Health, Mental Retardation, and Substance Abuse Services
Maine	Education		
Maryland	Education	Washington	Social and Health Services
Massachusetts	Public Health	West Virginia	Health and Human Resources
Michigan	Education	Wisconsin	Health and Family Services
Minnesota	Education	Wyoming	Health

National Early Childhood Technical Assistance Center, Chapel Hill, NC, reprinted with permission.

Through cooperative agreements with other agencies and independent providers, the lead agency assigns financial responsibilities of the program at the local level. The lead agency needs to have policies in place to handle inter- and intra-agency disputes, ensure that services are provided to infants and toddlers and their families in a timely manner and in the most natural environments possible, secure timely reimbursement of costs through funding under the program, compile data requested by the Secretary of Education, and advise and be advised by the state interagency coordinating council.

How Part C Services Are Funded

State grant allotments are prorated according to the comparative number of infants and toddlers with disabilities each state has, but the minimum amount is $500,000 a year. States must apply for these funds, and to be eligible, they must have statewide systems in place (administered by the interagency coordinating councils), as well as policies that provide for 0–3 intervention to all children with disabilities in the state. There is an outreach component to Part C that requires the lead agency to find these children through advertising campaigns and by other means.

The application must designate the lead agency, as well as the individual within it, responsible for assigning financial responsibility among appropriate agencies.

The application must also list a description of services that will be offered, including those to at-risk children, a description of the uses to which federal aid will be put, a description of how the program will guarantee distribution to all areas of the state, and assurance of public hearings and the opportunity for public comment before policies are adopted.

Defining Best Practice

Although government-funded early intervention has been helping infants and toddlers and their families for more than a decade, "best practice" in early intervention remains a nebulous goal. Early intervention involves different kinds of outcomes—parenting competencies, child development, educational readiness, and cost reduction—all of which are supposed to be pursued simultaneously. Furthermore, EI practice includes many professions, each of which has its own focus and methodology. Because of the diversity of goals and professions involved, it is more useful to speak about best *practices* in EI. Although EI programs differ widely, the most successful programs include cross-training of personnel where it is possible and focus on achieving a clearly defined set of positive outcomes for children and families. The many providers involved in EI approach intervention from within the basic philosophies of their own disciplines or from various schools of social science; however, early intervention administrators, clinicians, and program evaluators agree that the most important factor in success is a solid relationship between the provider and the family.

In February 2005, the Early Childhood Outcomes Center, a research and development arm of the federal Office of Special Education Programs (OSEP) put out the first defined report, *Family and Child Outcomes for Early Intervention and Early Childhood Special Education*, on what the basic outcomes in early intervention should be. The report is based on preliminary data from EI programs around the country. One of the ideas behind the report is to introduce accountability standards into future reauthorizations of IDEA and to lay the foundation for developing measurable results in early intervention that states can adopt. There are eight suggested outcomes—five for families using EI, preschool, and school-based services, and three for their children.

Family Outcomes

1. Families understand their children's strengths, abilities, and special needs.

2. Families know their rights and effectively communicate their children's needs.

3. Families help their children develop and learn.

4. Families feel they have adequate social support.

5. Families are able to access services and activities that are available to all families in their communities.

Children's Outcomes

1. Children have positive social relationships.

2. Children acquire and use knowledge and skills.

3. Children take appropriate actions to meet their needs.

It is also important to determine what a family's specific priorities are for their child and how those goals can be realistically accomplished. Occupational therapy in EI centers on the child and the therapist participating in tasks together. A successful EI therapist must teach family members how to care for and interact with their child as they participate in the child's treatment sessions. Occupational therapists will be familiar with how activity-based approaches can open closed doors, as activities become symbolic keys to the heart and mind. As you interact with your young clients, their parents should be watching, listening, and thinking. The best scenario to have in home-based EI is for at least one parent to take part in the session. He or she practices, with your active involvement, more ways to stimulate, motivate, and connect with the child. The parenting skills developed in these sessions carry over when you are not present.

Creating a Model of Care

If you make the principles of best practice discussed above your priorities, there is a real opportunity for you to create your own model of care for EI. Creating a model of care is not unlike putting together a professional development plan, but this model needs to center on the home environment and the roles of the people you will be encountering there. To succeed, you must be willing to become an expert on infancy and early childhood in your field. Consider getting more education on aspects of pediatric care with which you are unfamiliar, either formally or informally. The following steps will help you create the skill foundation needed for best practice in early intervention.

- Read and become familiar with the latest reauthorization of IDEA. Use it to create a mission statement for your practice, built around the law's intent. You can find Part C on the Internet at numerous sites. Print it out and study it thoughtfully. If you do, you will see that it encourages the kind of intervention you would like to give (i.e., occupational and psychosocial care in the child's natural environment).

- Highlight the parts of the law that pertain to the things you think are most important. The law may become your best ally as a provider if you learn it well. Remember that the purpose of IDEA is to help children with disabilities and their parents live well together and to solve or prevent problems that may create issues later on in school.

- If you are not using yourself as a therapeutic tool in your sessions, begin now. In the case at the beginning of this chapter, Susan redirected a mother's unrealistic vision of her child's future by responding therapeutically to the mother's unexpected question with insightful humor. This is called therapeutic use of self; it is psychosocial intervention. You must be able to trust and use this skill if you want to succeed in the home environment. You will need it to motivate, to evaluate the dynamics of the circumstances you encounter, and to facilitate successful role performance in a home disrupted by catastrophe. If you need more psychology training, get it.

- Educate yourself in normal childhood behavior patterns. Typical children and their parents sometimes find it hard to deal with one another, so you can imagine the behavioral issues that arise when parents are dealing with a child they may be afraid to discipline, especially at a time when the child needs those limits most. You need to be able to differentiate inappropriate behavior from pathology.

- Communicate. You are not in this alone, and you will not succeed alone. You must be able to deal with all kinds of people: case managers, agency heads, other EI personnel, and family members. Model your family-inclusive approach to other therapists when you can, and make your philosophy clear to your superiors. Educate them on the law if necessary. They may be so bogged down in red tape that they have forgotten the law's true intent regarding family involvement. Be willing to go out on a limb to remind them of the centrality of the family to EI if necessary.

Confronting Difficulties In Early Intervention Practice

Most agencies have their patients' best interests at heart, but the spirit of IDEA and the letter of it can differ significantly. Too often, the family aspect of treatment takes a back seat. Agencies sometimes operate as in-home care, forgetting that children in EI are there because they need certain kinds of attention from their parents, who must be taught these skills. Ask to see your agency's mission statement. It should be aligned with the intent of IDEA. If you see a need for improvement, you can then discuss it in terms of the law.

Agencies often assign certain therapists to evaluate and others to treat, creating an immediate middleman situation. Some do not make an effort to unify their treatment teams or to keep them in communication with one another. Many want to put anyone who comes through their door in treatment, because it is guaranteed income. They may hire inexperienced therapists who are not ready to work without supervision. If you find yourself working for an agency that wants to put money first, to the point of jeopardizing your best judgments and care, leave. Find another employer. It is that simple.

FOOD FOR THOUGHT

- How does IDEA try, in practice, to:
  - make sure a child gets the most efficient and effective intervention that he needs?
  - protect a child from abuse or neglect?
  - help parents be successful in helping their child?
- What things about the setting might discourage you from practicing in early intervention? In what way might you address or solve these problems?
- What roles do you play in the lives of your clients? Describe a situation in which you might be called upon to act as a facilitator.

Gestation, Birth, and Beyond

2

LIVING WITH DIFFICULT CHOICES: TWO VIEWS

Sally's Story

Jenny was in corporate sales; her husband, Dan, was a broker on Wall Street. They were in their middle 30s, and it had taken them two years to conceive a child. They named their daughter Sally as soon as the ultrasound revealed her sex. Soon after, a second sonogram indicated that Sally's head size was in the lowest range and the doctors feared she might have microcephaly.

Jenny had an amniocentesis, which revealed a chromosomal defect—an untreatable genetic abnormality. Hydrocephalus also was present, and the doctors explained that shortly after birth, they could insert a shunt to drain the fluid from her brain and relieve the pressure, or, because Sally would likely be born with significant birth defects, Jenny could terminate the pregnancy.

Jenny and Dan wanted their little girl and decided to pursue whatever treatment she would need at birth. At 7.5 months gestation, Jenny's water broke, and Sally was born 6 weeks early. Doctors resuscitated the baby, who was taken to the neonatal ICU. She stayed there for 8 weeks. She was fed through a gastric tube because her stomach and esophagus were not connected. She had anomalies of the face, ears, and hands and dysplasia of the hips. She could hear, and she was not blind. Her parents were given careful instructions about caring for her and did so attentively. EI provided services to stimulate senses and avoid contractures. Sally's parents envisioned a happy life for their daughter, despite her disabilities, and they often spoke about how thankful they were that she had been born.

Tarif's Story

Tarif was born to Adamu and Lami, new immigrants from Nigeria, both of whom were physicians. They both worked at a major hospital where Lami received excellent prenatal care. There was not one indication of a problem during her entire pregnancy. Tarif was full term, but problems with vaginal delivery caused fetal distress, and his heart stopped beating. A rapid C-section saved his life, but the umbilical cord had strangled him, and he had swallowed meconium. Immediately after birth, his Apgar score was zero. The medical staff resuscitated him and sent him to neonatal ICU. He had no anomalies, but he was blind and severely brain damaged. His swallow reflex was absent, and he had to be fed through a tube.

At 6 weeks, Tarif went home. His parents wept as they struggled to care for an infant who screamed at the slightest touch. Overwhelmed and unable to accept their severely handicapped child, they considered sending him to Nigeria to be cared for by their extended family. After the second visit, Tarif's parents discontinued EI services, because they concluded that therapy offered no hope for him. They chose simply to have a nurse follow the case instead.

Children are living today with birth defects that would have taken their lives 20 years ago. You will see some of them in early intervention, and they will be your most difficult cases. Their parents have had to make agonizing choices and face untold heartache. Your job is to teach those parents how to meet their newborns' needs, but the parents will ultimately decide what those needs are.

Remember when you come into a home and see a mother-child relationship, you are seeing not just the outer trappings of that bond—what is going on now—but all of the things that went before (the mother's response to the pregnancy itself, her shock in learning that her infant would be disabled or her surprise at the disability at birth, and her struggle to find a place in her mind for this child after birth) and all that the mother desperately hopes will follow.

Keeping the context of the pregnancy and birth in mind will help you to empathize with the parents of the children you serve. This can help you reach an agreement on priorities for the child and open a dialogue with the family. This dialogue should strengthen the parents and make them feel that they are capable of learning the skills they need to help their child. It will also focus their thoughts on the tasks at hand and away from the fear of the unknown. Kindness and honesty from you will build their trust.

When you are working with children who have life-altering disabilities, you too, need a personal perspective about these situations that can carry you through the most heart-wrenching cases. Build a sustaining personal philosophy that can help you to deal with the suffering of children with severe disabilities and their families and to focus on all of their needs. In the face of despair, you must preserve your own positive attitude.

An Overview of Human Development

The amazing thing about the human development process is that the blueprint actually becomes the final product. Perhaps more amazing is that a baby's developing systems begin working long before birth, so that a fetus actually urinates inside the gestational sac by the third month of pregnancy. At 25 days—often before the mother even knows she is pregnant—the fetal heart is pumping blood, although the heartbeat cannot yet be heard through a stethoscope.

Because of the mapping of the human genome, we now know how the human sperm and egg use the directions inside them to create a living creature. The penetration of the ovum by the sperm closes a door. Immediately the egg creates a charge (fence) around it that will keep out any other sperm. It will take about 12 hours for the pronucleus of the sperm, with its 23 chromosomes, to reach the pronucleus of the egg, with its 23 chromosomes. In about two hours they will fuse, and then, in another 18 hours, this 46-chromosome nucleus will divide into two cells, and then into three. By the three-celled stage, some scientists now believe, the "decision" whether to stay single or divide into identical twins has been made (Jones & Schraeder, 1987).

Chromosomal Abnormalities

In the vast majority of full-term pregnancies, the chromosomes are genetically intact. When there is a change or mutation in one or more chromosome, there is a high possibility of damage to the structural integrity and functionality of the body. In one type of chromosomal error, there are three copies of a certain chromosome present instead of the normal two, a situation called a trisomy. It is probable that very few fetuses with chromosomal abnormalities survive gestation since studies suggest that as many as 50 percent of all very early pregnancies end in miscarriage before the mother even knows she is pregnant (Wilcox et al., 1998). A fetus's chromosomal count is detectable by amniocentesis, a common test for at-risk pregnancies, which draws a sample of the mother's amniotic fluid directly from the sac during the second trimester of pregnancy. If chromosomal mutation disrupts the formation of the head, brain, or other vital organs, the risk of miscarriage, still birth, or death shortly after birth is high. Even in cases where the child survives, he or she is likely to require some level of special care throughout life.

Other Problems in Utero

Not all birth defects are chromosomal. Some, like cerebral palsy (CP), happen because of damage to the fetus in the uterus or during birth. CP was long believed to be the product of a birth injury, in which the infant suffered hypoxia in the birth canal, but new research strongly indicates that a virus in the mother's bloodstream is responsible for CP (Batshaw, 2002).

Other problems may become apparent at any time during pregnancy via blood tests, ultrasound, and radiography as the embryo grows into a fully developed fetus. Some abnormalities, including certain heart problems, are surgically correctable in utero. Other birth defects are not correctable or may not manifest until after birth. For further discussion see Chapter 6.

Pregnancy Culture

Though a pregnancy is usually detected within about 8 weeks of conception, if not before, it can take another month for a woman to settle into her pregnant state, and up to four months for the father to begin to prepare for this change in his life. Fathers are often unable to fully envision the coming birth until the pregnancy shows.

There are few studies of comparative culture in pregnancy, but those that exist note that transition to parenthood is a challenge for new parents with each child. Both mother and fetus can suffer negative consequences from stress during this period.

Was the pregnancy unwanted or unintended? If so, there is likely to be a delay in seeking prenatal care, a higher risk of domestic violence against the mother, a higher frequency of depression, a negative attitude toward the baby, and possibly even abuse (Orr, Miller, James, & Babones, 2000). In the United States, about 31 percent of all pregnancies resulting in a live birth are unintended. They are not necessarily *unwanted*, however. The numbers of unplanned pregnancies vary by marital status and ethnic group. In one study, 60 percent of unmarried women said their pregnancies were unintended (Abma et al., 1997 [as cited in Maldonado, 2003]); that number rose to 83 percent for unmarried African American women. About 39 percent of unmarried Latino women said their pregnancies were not planned (Peacock et al., 2000 [as cited in Maldonado, 2003]).

What an unplanned pregnancy means to a prospective mom depends entirely on her perspective, the timing of the event, her relationship with the baby's father and other significant people in her life, and the values of her family.

How Values Affect Pregnancy

Many sociologists agree that no matter where it happens around the world, a pregnancy that is welcomed is commonly regarded with hope. That is, the wish for the baby to be born healthy is shared by people from many diverse backgrounds. There is also a common fear of the outcome for mother and child that each culture handles differently, through rituals, habits, or customs that are embedded within that culture's values and are meant to protect mother and child. Virtually every family you see will have a lifestyle that exists in the context of cultural and sub-cultural realities, whether those are founded in ethnicity, economics, or demographics. The parents' background, how they make their living, and where they live greatly influence what they consider meaningful in terms of raising their baby. If you look and listen carefully, they will communicate these things to you as you visit them in their home. Other people in their lives also participate in these feelings and activities, and you will deal with some of them: grandparents, aunts, uncles, and the siblings of the child you are treating.

If the child you are seeing is an infant, a mother often wants to re-tell the story of her pregnancy, and may even refer to something that she felt was "not right" or "different" about it, as she tries to find a way to understand a newborn's health issues. Encourage this discussion if she begins it because it will help you to form a therapeutic bond with the mom that will increase her trust in you.

J. Martin Maldonado-Duran, a Topeka, Kansas, physician and principal investigator for the child and family center at Menninger Clinic in Houston, Texas, has studied and compared different cultural approaches to pregnancy.

He says that cultural customs and taboos reflect the social and economic realities of a society or neighborhood. In general, people in the lower socioeconomic social strata in the United States take a view of pregnancy similar to those in the same economic strata around the world. Pregnancy is viewed as a natural consequence, and women do not expect to fully control what happens to their bodies: a baby is considered the decision of a higher power. Having children is considered to be a duty of married women, and families welcome children regardless of the circumstances in which they enter the world (Maldonado, 2003).

Such a philosophy accommodates the lack of control people of lower socioeconomic status often feel they have over their lives, and it builds faith for strength in hard times. In societies or neighborhoods that are more affluent and have higher education levels, such views are sometimes considered archaic. Women are responsible not only for bearing children, but also for bearing them *at the right time*, when the family is prepared financially and emotionally (Maldonado, 2003).

Nevertheless, unwed teen mothers in homes of any ethnic background are likely to experience parental disapproval to varying degrees. With or without having told their parents about their circumstances, they may decide that they are on their own and must make their decisions about what to do independently, with little or no support. These are the cases that sometimes end in late-term abortions, self-mutilation, secret deliveries, and abandoned newborns you hear about on the news.

Dealing With Maternal Rejection

Few mothers are going to come right out and say, "I don't want this child," although you will find a few who might come close once they get to know you. There are a number of signs of rejection, but what is most essential is the prevention of any abuse that might come from rejection. Is the mother disinterested in the baby? Does she sit passively and not pay attention to the session? Is her treatment of the child indifferent, haphazard, or rough? A mother who is angry with the infant or toddler's father for his desertion of her can easily project those feelings on to the child. You cannot restore a relationship between parents that is over, but you can help the family through difficult circumstances.

Your first priority is to make sure that the child is safe. If the mother is negligent of the child's health or safety, make it clear that you are seeing something that is illegal, and that you will have to report it to the case manager. If there is not negligence at this point, but the child is clearly at risk for it, speak to the mother about specific things she needs to do: "You need to be really careful that your son doesn't get hurt." Or tell her: "Your daughter needs to have three meals each day, with nourishing food such as whole grains, lean meat or fish, dairy products like milk or cheese, and fresh fruits and vegetables."

Mothers of children with autistic disorders, in particular, are often highly frustrated because they find it difficult to connect with their children because of the children's lack of eye contact or verbalization, their repetitive/obsessive behaviors, and/or their tactile defensiveness and sporadic aggressiveness. If a child has been diagnosed as being on the autism spectrum, agencies sometimes use an interdisciplinary approach to treatment, introducing the child to several members of the team to see which of them might elicit the most positive response. That individual then becomes the primary therapist on the case. This requires some interdisciplinary training, however. Other team members rely on that individual to keep track of their respective concerns and give the treating therapist tips on how to handle those concerns.

Finding the best way to communicate with the child is the most important issue in defusing parental helplessness and frustration. Various disciplines have developed different ways of doing this, and the Autism Society of America lists these on its Web site (www.autism-society.org) under "treatment," then "learning approaches," explaining each approach and discussing its strengths and weaknesses.

Occupational therapists treat this disorder as a sensory-processing issue, and therefore, attend to sensory deficits, concentrating a great deal on vestibular stimulation and tactile desensitizing. But these are not their only purview.

Two approaches the Autism Society suggests that would work well in the 0–3 population are the Picture Exchange Communication System (PECS) developed by the Delaware Autistic Program, in which the child can chose a picture to tell how he or she is feeling or what her or she is thinking; and Floor Time, an educational model developed by child psychiatrist Stanley Greenspan that encourages general playtime among parent, therapist, and child to let the child take the lead in directing action, but working on developmental goals together.

Both of these techniques were born out of applied behavioral analysis (ABA), one of the most used, and yet controversial, techniques applied in autism treatment today. In ABA a psychologist, or another person trained in the therapy, uses an action-response approach to try to change problematic behaviors by breaking them down into small tasks, for which the child is rewarded with something he or she likes when he or she accomplishes them.

ABA requires intense work with the child in what some people feel is too rote a way of teaching. The Cambridge Center for Behavioral Studies (CCBS) in Concord, Massachusetts, (www.behavior.org) offers a full explanation of this approach, when it works best and with whom, and how to make sure the practitioner using it is qualified.

Putting some distance between parent and child is always an option when it seems that neglect or abuse is a risk or when the parent's frustration level has reached its limit. Discuss with your agency or case manager the option of putting the child in center-based EI instead of treating the child in the home. If the case manager tells you the option is available, you can make the suggestion to the parent.

Summary

Even within marriage, pregnancy is a vulnerable time for a woman. Every culture and subculture has management rules for pregnancy. They are do's and don'ts that are meant to protect mother and infant. You might hear them referred to as "old wives' tales." They are based in cultural experience, not medical knowledge, and they are very important to the families you will see. The cultural setting of the pregnancy will greatly affect the environment into which the baby is born—whether the child will live with one other person or several, in poverty or wealth, with open affection or reserve, with industriousness or apathy, and with values that are compatible or incompatible with mainstream ethics. Each set of people and circumstances you meet is unique. Learning to observe, listen, and ask the right questions will tell you a great deal about the family with whom you are dealing.

FOOD FOR THOUGHT

- Examine your own philosophy of life. What do you value about it? How do you handle unexpected or tragic circumstances?

- Have you found that your own cultural background helps or hinders you in connecting with people who are different from you? Factors to consider include ethnic groups different from your own, higher or lower socioeconomic status, and higher or lower levels of education. How might that affect your work in EI?

- What type of behavior might signal that a mother feels uncomfortable with her child's disability?

Working With the Family

3

CHARLIE'S STORY

Charlie was 18 months old. He was put in EI because he was easily fatigued and the distal phalangeal joints of his ring and little fingers were slightly spastic and had started to rest in flexion. There was concern about them becoming permanently contracted and interfering with fine-motor function in the future.

Charlie had a stay-at-home mom, an 8-month old sister, and a 3-year-old brother named Billy. I scheduled my session during the baby's naptime, but Billy was always there and wanted to play too. When there is a sibling too young to fully understand that his brother or sister needs special help, it is often best to administer small group treatment and create and support therapeutic play involving both of them. Otherwise, you risk the possibility of creating jealously, envy, and attention-getting behavior, ranging from tears to temper tantrums.

Because Charlie was the younger child and was developmentally behind, it was easy to involve Billy in a big-brother helping role. I gave them each a bit of dough to roll into snakes and pinch into pieces. If Billy understood something Charlie did not, I would show Billy how to tell or show Charlie. You could see his pride as he helped his brother. He learned how to work with Charlie hand-over-hand, gently pressing down on his fingers to stretch them. He learned to hand over tiny objects so Charlie had to use his ring and little fingers only to grasp them.

Charlie had the most patience of any child his age I have ever treated. He would try over and over to pick a tiny object up in thumb-ring or thumb-little finger opposition. Billy would show him how to handle a particular object then cheer Charlie on. "You can do it Charlie. I know you can. WOW! You did it! You did it!"

Charlie's mother learned to passively stretch the joints throughout the day. We told Billy that it was a Mommy job, and he understood. The mother bought some dough to use when I was not there and put together a box full of small, variously shaped objects. She said Billy usually played therapeutically with Charlie indoors, because he fatigued less quickly that way. The boys had also become closer.

When I walked into their home, the two little boys would run up and hug my legs, and I would pick each up and hug them. Billy never knew I was primarily there to see Charlie; I came to see them both. Therapy ended after 8 sessions because the family had learned the skills necessary to help Charlie themselves. For that reason, I did not get to know the family as well as others I have worked with. I was very surprised when I was shopping a couple of months later and I heard a small voice yell, "Dr. Ja-a-a-ane!" A quarter of the way across the store, waving from the child's seat in the basket, was Billy. I went over and hugged him. "I miss you," I said. "I miss you, too," he answered. Then he pointed down to Charlie, napping in the basket, "And Charlie does, too."

What Is a Family?

We are going to assume in this chapter that the home consists of a mother, a father, and siblings. You may work with any or all of them, but your goal is to have them work together when you are done.

What if the home is not a traditional one, and the people there are related in various ways or some are not related at all? (You will see many households like this.) Is this a family? Not legally, perhaps, but the public concept of "family" in the United States today seems to be changing from those people related by blood or marriage to whoever shares the same household and takes responsibility for each other's welfare. This is happening because mothers and fathers are often split by divorce or other circumstances, and they may live with their own parents, other relatives, or friends.

Of course, as far as the infant is concerned, family is whoever takes care of his or her needs and gives him or her love and affection. These are the people who spend the most time with the infant. They are the people with whom you will work in the home.

Infants from all ranges of socioeconomic strata may have caregivers other than their mothers. Higher income families may have nannies who raise the children on a full-time basis. Lower income families must often leave them in center-based care, with babysitters or relatives who come to the parents' home during working hours, or who care for the child in their own homes.

Household Roles

Children develop their sense of self through feedback from other family members. As they grow, they continue to see themselves partly through this mirror and adapt in whatever ways are necessary to get their needs met. They will establish their own identity within the family unit.

The key for siblings to safely assimilate a new birth is to know they have not lost their value to their parents. Young children need to be reassured by word and deed that they are still loved just as much as they ever were and that they will continue to be loved. Older children also need to feel important—a necessary part of the adjustment process. Communication of thoughts and feelings, offered with some degree of sensitivity, is of paramount importance in families, and each member must learn to respect the feelings of others even if he or she does not share those feelings. Talking honestly opens the door to understanding (Tucker-Ladd, 1996).

As you read about role-playing within the family, envision how the situation would change if the new baby had a chronic illness or disability that would last his whole life.

Mom and Dad

Even if they enjoyed a non-traditional lifestyle before the baby was born, both partners are likely to take up more traditional roles when they become parents. Becoming a mother is a profound change in a woman's life. If she is secure in her relationship with the baby's father, and he is living in the home, she may have a tendency to put him second. The baby's needs are so great that for the first few weeks, everyone's life centers on the infant. Instead of two adults sharing their lives, the couple is now a family devoting their attention to the baby. Mothers usually find fulfillment in this, but fathers often do not. The father may feel shut out of the baby's life, especially if the mother is breastfeeding. He might like to be a hands-on father, but may not be encouraged to be one (Tucker-Ladd, 1996).

A mother may not be able to give her husband as much time or attention as she did before the baby arrived, and the father may experience feelings of resentment towards the baby. Just like the siblings, the father needs to know his wife still values him as much as she did before the baby was born. Mothers should not dismiss this as childish, as these feelings are very common. If this is not the first child, the father is often surprised to find himself in charge of the older children while the mother tends to the baby. If he is close to them, this transition is not a problem, but if he paid only minimal attention to his older children until now, he may be at a loss when it comes to taking care of their needs.

Both parents will go without adequate sleep for at least a few weeks, and if the baby is not a good sleeper, sleep deprivation can wreak havoc in the household. Tempers flare, tears flow, and home seems anything but a haven from the world. If the mother suffers any degree of post-partum depression, the situation becomes even more stressful.

SHE LOVES ME, SHE LOVES ME NOT...

By Jill Diffendal

Many Americans had never paid attention to the term "postpartum depression" until Texas mother Andrea Yates murdered her five children in June 2001.

And coverage of Yates' case, which ended in a life sentence for her, and others like it are a "mixed bag" for the cause of public awareness, according to Karen Kleiman, MSW, an author and expert on postpartum disorders.

"[These cases have] absolutely increased the awareness of health care practitioners," said Kleiman, who in 1988 founded the Postpartum Stress Center in Bryn Mawr, PA. "But in terms of the women themselves, it has had a reverse effect. It is scaring them into greater silence. If they tell someone about their symptoms, they worry, 'Are they going to take my baby away?' The media did a disservice to the cause because they didn't define the parameters well—they called it postpartum depression when it was not. It was a complete psychotic episode."

Postpartum psychosis affects one to two out of 1,000 women and constitutes a "life-threatening medical emergency [that] requires immediate medical attention," said Diana Lynn Barnes, PsyD, MFT, licensed marriage and family therapist and founder of the Center for Postpartum Health in Woodland Hills, CA.

As many as four out of five mothers experience what has been traditionally called the baby blues; symptoms will diminish within two weeks with added reassurance, support and rest for the new mom. Between the two falls postpartum depression (PPD), often used as an umbrella term for postpartum stress syndrome, postpartum anxiety/panic disorder and postpartum obsessive-compulsive disorder. Experts estimate that PPD effects 10 to 20 percent of mothers.

(continued)

What Is Normal?

"There is nothing fancy about the term 'postpartum depression'—it is a clinical depression in the postpartum period," said Kleiman. "For the most part, postpartum depression really presents in many ways identical to general depression [although] it can present differently and be identified as anxiety. The biggest difference is, we have a baby in the picture, so it can be more dramatic in the sense that there is the impact of the baby on mom in addition to her being depressed. And frequently there is more of an urgency to recover."

PPD is often not identified because women don't understand the difference between the baby blues and more serious postpartum disorders. According to Barnes, it is "normal" for women to expect to feel exhausted, tearful, moody, anxious, impatient, irritable, restless and let down.

"Their body has gone through a tremendous amount, and their hormones are out of whack," Barnes said frankly. "The baby blues usually crop up around day 3, and by day 14 women will generally even out. But if these symptoms begin to exacerbate or persist—if they are interfering with her functioning—then it is not normal. Usually in postpartum depression it is as though the body shuts down. When a mother feels this way, it has to be honored and listened to."

PPD can affect mothers up to a year after childbirth. As a mother moves into the realm of PPD, she may feel like she is unable to cope, have difficulty sleeping despite exhaustion, or experience significant changes in eating habits. She may feel detached from her infant. She may experience intrusive thoughts, feelings of guilt, confusion, hopelessness, inadequacy, disinterest or fear of losing control. Women with postpartum depression are at high risk for suicidal thoughts, but they often express it in different ways.

"Most women may not say directly that they want to kill themselves, but they may talk about feeling trapped or hoping for some type of accident so they can be taken away from all of their pain," Barnes added.

Risk Factors

Alerting women to what is normal and what is PPD is half the battle; the other half requires that health care practitioners learn more about symptoms and risk factors for PPD.

"One of the complaints I get is that [these women] are not being listened to," said Barnes. "They go to a doctor and say 'I feel weird' or 'I can't stop crying.' But the doctor may say 'Well, you are just adjusting.' So we go home and we say '[The doctor] must know,' and we sit for months with these symptoms."

Understanding the risk factors may encourage health care practitioners to identify women at risk and set up a prevention plan. Barnes classifies risk factors into three categories: biological, environmental and psychological. Biological risk factors include a previous experience with postpartum depression; a personal or family history of depression, mood disorders or thyroid conditions; or very long or short intervals between pregnancies. History of bipolar disorders or schizophrenia puts women at higher risk for postpartum psychosis.

(continued)

A woman with psychological risk factors may have had a strained or ambivalent relationship with her own mother. Barnes explained that "a woman who may have a conflicted or ambivalent relationship with her own mother may come to motherhood and say 'I don't know what it means to be a good mother.'" The severe physiological and psychological stress of childbirth may reactivate early trauma from sexual, verbal or physical abuse. Chemical dependency is also a psychological risk factor.

Environmental factors that put woman at risk for PPD include a complicated pregnancy or delivery, a Caesarian section, a premature birth or a colicky or otherwise unhealthy infant. Fertility issues are an environmental factor but can also become a psychological factor if the woman feels pressured to conceive and a biological factor if fertility drugs are used. Marital conflict and lack of a good support system are high on the list of external factors. Stressors in other areas, such as a move or financial issues, also place women at higher risk.

On top of these risk factors, many women bring more stress on themselves because "we are not very good at taking care of ourselves," said Barnes, who herself endured an episode of PPD 10 years ago. New mothers often deprive themselves of sleep, proper nutrition and relaxation, all of which place them at higher risk for anxiety and depression.

Interestingly, in Kleiman's experience, mothers of infants born with disabilities or chronic health conditions do not appear to be at higher risk for PPD. "Women with a NICU baby are often referred to me by an adjunctive health care professional," she said, stressing that this has been her own experience only. "Women who are distracted by the health of their baby don't feel like they have the luxury to feel bad. They feel like they are justified, they have a 'reason' to be depressed."

According to Kleiman, understanding risk factors and symptoms may not be enough, because many women experiencing PPD are very good at hiding the symptoms.

"We live in a culture that doesn't really tolerate mothers not feeling good," she explained. "It is scary to say out loud 'I am feeling something that is not so great,' so women hide and isolate and hope it goes away." To thwart this phenomenon, Kleiman advocates a protocol for screening all mothers around six weeks postpartum. "Doctors should have that information," she added. "They are letting women out of their offices who are at tremendous risk."

Treating the Problem

Once a woman has been diagnosed with PPD, treatment options can vary depending on the factors involved. The mother should undergo a medical exam to rule out physiological causes, especially thyroid dysfunction since as many as 10 percent of new mothers will develop thyroid problems after childbirth. A psychiatric evaluation, preferably by a professional familiar with postpartum disorders, will identify appropriate therapeutic interventions, generally psychotherapy and/or psychoactive medications. Most PPD advocates also stress the value of participation in support groups.

(continued)

"The most important thing for women who are experiencing a mood disorder is to create some sense of safety for themselves because this is a very scary time when you need all your physical and emotional stamina," Barnes said. "It is not always just about slipping someone some Prozac. We know the best prognosis is a combination of therapy and medication with adjuncts like group support."

For occupational therapists dealing with new mothers, postpartum depression is rarely a topic of discussion. OTs can, however, encourage awareness and direct troubled mothers to seek appropriate help.

"You can ask very basic questions—Are you overwhelmed? Are you feeling sad a lot of the time? How does it feel to have this baby?—and create the opportunity for her to respond," Kleiman said. "The best thing an adjunctive practitioner can do is let a mother know that it is not normal to feel bad for four months. We need to make it OK for women to admit that they don't feel so good. If we are treating her or her child for something else, then that, too, is part of the postpartum picture."

On a grander scale, creating that safe environment is a societal issue. "As a culture we really romanticize childbirth," Barnes cautioned. "We don't account for the stresses that life cycle change brings to the family. Implied in these changes is an enormous amount of loss: loss of routine, time, schedule, adult companionship, romantic relationship with your partner. We tell women that you are going to know exactly what to do and it will be love at first sight; but when women experience discrepancies with what we tell them, they suffer in silence and put themselves at risk."

Combating PPD also needs to be a family-centered process, especially since the father's role in and reaction to PPD is often overlooked. Men need to feel comfortable with expressing themselves and be encouraged to seek out appropriate outlets for their stress. After all, Barnes said, postpartum depression creates enormous tension in families. In her practice, she encourages couples to come see her together at least once to ensure that everyone has an opportunity to talk about their experience.

"This is truly a developmental crisis in the life cycle of the family," Barnes concluded. "What we need is a general overall campaign to educate people about this illness. We are still in the dark ages about depression and mood disorders. We don't recognize that postpartum depression is a biological illness caused by changes in brain chemistry brought about by childbirth."

From ADVANCE for Occupational Therapy Practitioners, Aug. 26, 2002. *Reprinted with permission.*

Brothers and Sisters

Siblings in the household will react to a new baby according to their ages and degrees of maturity. Each new child is not only a future playmate, but also a contender for what children feel is a limited amount of affection their parents have to offer. The situation has been compared to a love triangle: When mom and dad walk in the door with a new baby, their toddlers may feel the same way one parent would feel if the other brought home a lover. This analogy makes it easy to understand the intensity of the feelings at work. A very young sibling, with less developed language skills, is more apt to show anger at the new arrival. The anger is also mixed with affection, and the more the older child is allowed to safely interact with the baby, the easier things will be.

The older child is now a brother or sister. This is a new role to play, and one that will evolve over time. Some first-born children in large families have major responsibilities when it comes to keeping the home running smoothly during a new birth transition. These children may find themselves acting as surrogate parents to other siblings. Depending on the personality of the child, he or she may welcome this role and undertake it willingly. It is important that parents do not take advantage of this situation. Older siblings need time to be teenagers and to think about their own futures without falling into a caregiver pattern. The first-born in the family may be saddled with responsibility he or she did not ask for. Parents may treat their oldest child as the third adult in the household, expecting that individual to behave beyond the maturity level of his or her years.

Middle siblings may find themselves on their own for a time, because the parents cannot give them as much attention—or supervision—as they did before the birth. Pre-teens may feel a new sense of freedom and get used to making more of their own decisions. When the baby is settled in, parents are likely to return their attention to their other children, and a battle may ensue. Young siblings, those who are still toddlers, may regress and become more babyish for a while. They may suddenly "forget" their toilet training and may want their parents to do things for them that they have done for themselves for a long time.

If siblings are present in the home when you are there, encourage them to become part of the therapeutic process. Getting involved in the treatment process can make them more vital participants in family living. Infants with slightly older brothers and sisters (preschool age) usually enjoy interacting with them. Often, another child can hold the baby's attention better than an adult. The infant must be medically stable, of course, to ensure safety. With infants, visual tracking, strengthening arms and legs, gaining postural stability, crossing midline, crawling, cruising, and feeding are often part of the goals. Let the sibling watch you engage the baby, and then let them try it. This should not be a regular handling experience unless the sibling is on the floor, is being guarded, and has the parent's permission.

Children appreciate showing off their talents. Let them role model for the baby. Some disruptive siblings are really just looking to feel needed and important, because the baby is getting so much attention. With an infant, get older siblings (grade school age) into the act with the parents. This is family-centered treatment. You are teaching family members how to interact with one another as they accomplish something together.

If the child you are treating is a toddler, you have a lot more room to be creative. Toddlers have some skills and can communicate with older brothers and sisters. The two and three year olds want to achieve. They want to be able to say, "I did it!" Older siblings can often elicit better responses from the toddler than the parents. Children of any age seem to have an innate ability to communicate with each other. Have you ever watched a toddler trying to talk to a frustrated parent who just cannot understand him, only to have his 6-year-old sister walk into the room, listen, and accurately interpret his wishes?

Younger toddlers may be working on gross and fine motor skills, older toddlers on graphomotor skills and vestibular activities (e.g., balance, coordination, etc.). Even if the child you are treating needs a great deal of adaptive equipment, older brothers and sisters can be taught to facilitate it. They will also need to be taught to allow their younger sibling to do things independently. The family often forms a habit of doing too much for the child with a disability when coaching and encouragement are the best tools to use. Even if the child fails, family members should let him or her try it again and again. Children of all ages in the family learn patience and appreciation by getting involved in treatment.

Others in the Home

Some homes include grandparents, and you may work with them. Particularly in single-parent situations, the grandmother may become the live-in babysitter while her son or daughter goes back to work. A grandparent is often highly interested in the baby's care, and sometimes has more time to spend with the child. If you never seem to see the parents, however, make it clear to the caregiver that they need to find a way to get involved. Contact your agency if necessary. Both parents may be at work, but you need to involve them in some way.

You will see many kinds of dynamics among extended family members that you will count as productive or counter-productive to your treatment goals. Some cultures naturally live in large groups that include members of the extended family. Others prefer a small nuclear family unit. The household may be noisy, or people may be coming in and out while you are there. If you can identify what seems meaningful to this particular family unit quickly, you are far more likely to engender cooperation and success. Is there a religious holiday going on? Maybe you can incorporate some of their customs into your treatment. Is Uncle Sean a NASCAR nut? (Got some model cars?) Does Aunt Gina pride herself on her cooking? (Two- and three-year-olds can help in little ways.) Use whatever you can to tie that family unit together with your young patient.

Be careful to remember your place. You are not part of the family, and if your patient is only a few months old, you are arriving at a delicate time. The entrance of a new baby into the conjugal family increases the desire that family has for privacy. Their need for help may conflict with that desire. Remember that you are probably not the only discipline in the home. Therapists coming and going several times a week can add a great deal of stress to an already stressful time. Work with your team to determine who really needs to be there most, and allow that individual priority. If you are the one, be as flexible as possible in setting up your appointments. If you ignore this issue, you will often find people simply will not answer the door. They have their own ways of controlling their lives. If you have a constant problem with no-shows, ask honestly why it is happening before you discontinue working with the family.

The Disability Factor

In 1987, Emily Perl Kingsley, the mother of a son with Down syndrome, wrote an essay called *Welcome to Holland* that has been widely published, in which she described the "journey" of mothering a child with a disability:

> I am often asked to describe the experience of raising a child with a disability to try to help people who have not shared that unique experience to understand it, to imagine how it would feel. It's like this:

> When you're going to have a baby, it's like planning a fabulous vacation trip to Italy. You buy a bunch of guide books and make your wonderful plans: the Coliseum. Michelangelo's David. The gondolas in Venice. You may learn some handy phrases in Italian. It's all very exciting.

After months of eager anticipation, the day finally arrives. You pack your bags and off you go. Several hours later, the plane lands. The stewardess comes in and says, "Welcome to Holland."

"Holland?!" you say. "What do you mean Holland? I signed up for Italy! I'm supposed to be in Italy. All my life I've dreamed of going to Italy."

But there's been a change in the flight plan. They've landed in Holland and there you must stay.

The important thing is that they haven't taken you to a horrible, disgusting, filthy place, full of pestilence, famine and disease. It's just a different place.

So you must go out and buy new guide books. And you must learn a whole new language. And you will meet a whole new group of people you would never have met.

It's just a different place. It's slower-paced than Italy, less flashy than Italy. But after you've been there for a while and you catch your breath, you look around and you begin to notice that Holland has windmills—and Holland has tulips. Holland even has Rembrandts.

But everyone you know is busy coming and going from Italy... and they're all bragging about what a wonderful time they had there. And for the rest of your life, you will say "Yes, that's where I was supposed to go. That's what I had planned."

And the pain of that will never, ever, ever, ever go away, because the loss of that dream is a very, very significant loss. But if you spend your life mourning the fact that you didn't get to Italy, you may never be free to enjoy the very special, the very lovely things about Holland.

If the child is seriously ill but well enough to be cared for at home, it is likely that some of the patterns affecting spouses and siblings described above, usually temporary in the case of a healthy child, will become permanent. When a baby with a disability comes home, other children growing up in that home will find life as they knew it permanently changed. They will be required to adjust to their mother's new focus on the baby with special needs. Her personality may change. What should have been a joyous occasion has become one of sadness. The baby's siblings may be troubled by feelings of helplessness. If they are very young, they may hold themselves responsible for the younger sibling's disabilities, fearing something they said or did wrong caused it. Parents should be aware of this inner sense of guilt and assure their other children that they did nothing to cause this situation.

Older children and teenagers may question religious faith, angry that God will not answer their prayers to make the baby well. As children grow up with a sibling who has special needs, this anger usually dissipates. Siblings are likely to grow to love him or her a great deal and to protect this sibling at their own expense.

Raising a child with disabilities will become a family experience in which everyone in the household is likely to grow in maturity and understanding. Parents need to acknowledge the extra effort their child with special needs must put into his or her life process and support the child in this effort. Children with disabilities should be raised as much like their siblings as possible. It is often difficult for parents to teach discipline and reinforce behavior in their children with disabilities, but it is important that they do it.

It is very easy for children with disabilities to become self-absorbed. Their lives revolve around constant challenge. They must think about how to do the things that most people can do almost automatically. At school they sometimes have to endure the bullying of classmates. Life is about adapting to many different circumstances, and they reach for the tools they need—adaptive equipment, mobility aids, and sympathetic peers who fight for them or help them. It takes more effort for a child with a disability to learn empathy. Helping the child achieve this should be a family priority.

ON THE SIDELINES

By Jessica Alley

I don't remember thinking my sister was "different" when she came home as a newborn, though she was hooked to lots of wires as she slept in her new crib. I didn't know that it was to warn my parents of possible breathing abnormalities or even heart failure.

I don't even remember being told my sister had a life-threatening disease. I just knew.

I do remember the "sunshine packages" she always got during long stays at the hospital or while recovering at home in bed. Those packages had lots of beautifully wrapped gifts, all put together in one great big box. I hated those boxes. Not that my sister didn't share or even give some of the gifts to me, but the boxes were never addressed to me.

As the older sibling of a now young adult who was born with chronic intestinal pseudo-obstruction (CIP), a disease which makes her dependent on artificial support for nutrition and bladder control, I have only recently begun to realize that the feelings with which I grew up (and still occasionally wrestle) are completely normal. For the first time in my life, I am learning to let go of the guilt that builds up within me over jealousy or resentment I can't seem to control.

Do others in my circumstance feel this way? I needed to know, so I went looking for answers. What I found I believe will help both siblings and parents to understand the process by which we come to accept, live with and love our brothers and sisters with disabilities.

Concerns of Siblings

Among a number of organizations studying that process is Contact a Family (CAF), a United Kingdom charity that provides resources to families who care for children with disabilities or special needs. In polls conducted over the course of its existence, CAF discovered recurring themes in the dynamics of families with disabled or ill children. So CAF put together a fact sheet on the issues that siblings have raised about their lives with their disabled brothers and sisters.

(continued)

Limited Time and Attention From Parents

Many siblings feel jealous of the amount of attention their brothers and sisters receive. Because my sister was mostly home schooled, I always felt that I was missing out on activities that she and my mom shared while I was at school. I understood that the amount of time my parents spent with my sister versus the amount spent with me wasn't purposely unequal; it was something that couldn't be helped. But it was, and still is, hard at times.

Jennifer Dierkes, 28, remembers what it was like adjusting to the attention her brother received after his spinal cord injury. It was Memorial Day weekend 1989 when Matt Feeser, only a few days short of his 20th birthday, broke his neck at a water amusement park.

"He fell into a pool that was only about a foot deep," explained his sister. "He was leaning over the water to splash his face and lost his balance. He didn't realize how shallow the water was." Matt was left with quadriplegia.

That was 12 years ago. When she talked with ADVANCE about her brother, Dierkes said, "I honestly didn't have that feeling [of neglect from] my parents. I guess knowing that this was such a huge life change for my brother and parents, I didn't really take the lack of attention personally."

But Jennifer was a sophomore in high school at the time of Matt's accident, the same school where he had been a popular, outgoing student before graduating.

"When I would meet my teachers, the first question out of their mouth was 'How is your brother doing?' because they had heard of the accident, which is certainly understandable," said Dierkes. "But in the same respect, I was going through this massive life change as well, and I don't think I was ever really asked 'how are you doing?' That used to anger me...I felt like I could have been reached out to a little bit more."

CAF has suggestions for parents to meet the need for attention in their disabled children's siblings. Try setting aside certain times to spend with them alone, such as bedtime, or plan monthly outings or activities in order to have some one-on-one time together. If a disabled or ill child needs constant supervision, preparing ahead for short-term care can allow parents to attend important events of the other sibling, such as sports events and plays. Sometimes it is a good idea to put the needs of the able-bodied siblings first, advises CAF, even though it may be hard to do.

Why Her and Not Me?

During an International Pediatric Rheumatology Conference in Park City, UT, a few years ago, keynoter James May spoke about the impact of chronic illness and disability on the family. "[Siblings] experience guilt; their good health is in stark contrast to the special needs of their sibling," he explained. "Many siblings have been told they should not complain because they have been 'blessed with good health.'" From that point, it is easy to begin feeling guilt over one's own health.

Also, being reminded that I have opportunities that my sister doesn't has made me feel that I "got off lucky." I still feel some guilt over it.

(continued)

Dierkes said that because her brother's disability is the result of an accident, she often struggles with the question of "Why him and not someone else?"

"He had so much going for him," she said. "I often wonder where he would be right now if it hadn't happened…he would probably have a wife and kids."

CAF advises parents to emphasize that no one is to blame for the handicap and to encourage siblings to see their brothers or sisters as people with similarities and differences to themselves. Meeting other families who have children with similar conditions, perhaps through a support group, can help the siblings see that they are not alone in their feelings.

Love Me, Love Her

I have been very lucky in that my oldest friends have always taken my cue. My sister is part of the package: you take me and you get her, too. The difficulty is explaining her condition to new friends that come into my life. My sister appears to be a very normal, average girl. I haven't had to face the problems that siblings of severely handicapped children face.

Dierkes had to deal with friends questioning her brother's new lifestyle. Most of her friends during high school had also been a part of her childhood, so they had known her brother for a couple of years.

"I found that it wasn't that they didn't accept him," she explained. "But they had a lot of questions that they asked me because they were embarrassed to ask him, basic questions, like how he took care of himself."

CAF tells parents that they can help prepare their kids by talking over how to explain a brother or sister's difficulties to friends. The group also warns parents not to expect siblings to always include the child with special needs in their play or activities and, in the worst-case scenario, to invite friends around when the disabled child is away.

Stress at Home

Siblings that CAF surveyed said that they are often disturbed while sleeping and frequently feel tired at school. They also find it hard to complete homework.

I will never forget trying to explain to one high school teacher that my sister had been admitted to the hospital the night before, and I just wasn't able to concentrate on my homework assignment. Her response was that I had to learn not to use my sister's illness as an excuse in life. I was stunned. Not only did her words hurt, but I also wondered if she was right. Did I "use" my sister's illness as a way to get by situations I didn't want to deal with? This is a good example of when siblings need to talk to their parents. Only they could help me sort out the situation and reassure me that I did not take advantage of my sister, but instead was there for her.

Dierkes' brother's accident happened right before her finals at school, and she ended up failing most of them. She doesn't remember any of her teachers reassuring her that it was understandable to have difficulty preparing for and taking school tests during such a trying time in her and her family's life.

(continued)

The "family stress factors" section of the special-needs center at Smarterkids.com notes that some siblings take on more emotional stress than others. They may try to undertake the role of surrogate parent by assuming more responsibility than necessary, or try to compensate for the child with the disability by trying to make up for that child's limitations.

Parents need to encourage siblings to develop their own social lives, says CAF. It is important to try to keep a sense of humor in the family to ease stress. Parents should seek professional advice about how to include siblings in care-giving tasks and handling difficult behaviors. If privacy is an issue for a sibling with a brother or sister who has behavior problems, a lock on the bedroom door can prevent possessions from being damaged.

Restrictions on Family Activities

CAF found that siblings feel resentful when family outings are limited and infrequent. All events have to be carefully planned and all necessary precautions taken when it comes to a family with a disabled/ill child, and my family is no exception.

The hardest part is keeping in mind that any scheduled event always has the chance of being canceled at the last minute in the event that my sister gets sick. I just try to keep in mind that it is just as much of a disappointment to her and my parents as it is to me.

Dierkes agrees, saying that basic activities like going out to dinner are difficult for her family because so many places are actually not handicap accessible. She also had a hard time as a young adult accepting that her parents could no longer do the things they once did.

From ADVANCE for Occupational Therapy Practitioners, Oct. 15, 2001. *Reprinted with Permission.*

FOOD FOR THOUGHT

- How would you promote family involvement in a treatment situation when only the grandmother is home when you visit?

- The 30-month-old child you are treating has a 13-year-old brother who sometimes watches your treatment session. How would you encourage him to participate?

- The mother of the child you are seeing seems depressed. She is in her nightgown during sessions, and does not seem very responsive. She does not want to participate in the therapy session and would rather watch TV. How would you approach her to gain more information and cooperation?

Brain Development in Response to Experience

4

ABBY'S STORY

Abby's mother, Lisa, was in day treatment for schizophrenia; her father, Sean, had been laid off from his job doing light assembly work at a factory. He was taking care of Abby all day and her two older siblings after school. He was a shy, soft-spoken man who doted on Abby. At 24 months Abby was delayed in fine-motor skills and had been referred for occupational therapy. She was not completely weaned, had very little toilet training, was ill behaved, and threw frequent, uncontrollable temper tantrums. Sean tolerated her behavior because Abby had been an unplanned child. She was unwanted by her mother, who had developed psychotic postpartum depression.

When Sean and the occupational therapist were alone with her, Abby was quiet and cooperative. She enjoyed fine-motor activity and was fascinated by the crayons the OT had brought. Abby did not have her own crayons because Sean was afraid she might eat them or color inappropriate objects. The therapist explained to him that Abby needed to practice with the crayons between sessions and gave him a few in a baggie and a dozen sheets of paper so they could practice circles, squares, and triangles.

A few sessions later, Sean, Abby, and the therapist were working on the floor when Lisa entered the room. All of a sudden Abby began to crawl (she could and usually did walk) toward a corner of the room, screaming. She began to bite her hand. Lisa screamed at Abby, "Get your hand out of your mouth! Stop crying!" Abby looked toward her dad, screaming louder. Sean lowered his eyes, and Lisa stomped up the stairs to her bedroom. Sean picked up Abby, and she began to calm down.

The therapist called the service coordinator to request a provider meeting to discuss ways to address the dysfunctional relationships in the family. The coordinator explained that it would take some time to arrange such a meeting because the family had had 21 providers in the last few years! EI was providing a social worker, an OT, a speech therapist, a special education teacher, and a respite baby sitter. Other services provided home-based math and reading teachers and respite baby sitters to each of the older children. Adult services sent mental health counselors for the mother, the father, and the family. Then there were Social Security Aid to Dependent Children (AFDC), and child welfare counselors. They all came to the home. Lisa also had her own psychiatrist, counselor, and therapists at the day treatment center.

When the therapist asked Sean about the intervention overload, he smiled ruefully. "So many people are coming in—I feel I can't even breathe. But I'm afraid to say no because we need the checks. I'm afraid of losing my home and not being able to feed the kids." His wife was receiving Social Security Disability Income (SSDI) for her mental condition, and Sean believed that he had to accommodate any kind of help the family was offered in order to keep the money coming in.

The OT was amazed that any family could tolerate so much intervention. She told the service coordinator that Abby's delays seemed environmental, not physiological, and described Abby's response to her mother. She believed that the little girl would benefit by spending time away from home and suggested that occupational therapy at Head Start would be more appropriate than continuing OT at home.

Disability—in this case the mother's—almost always creates an unbalanced lifestyle in the family. Roles are disrupted as adults and children take on duties that prevent them from fulfilling their own needs. The dynamics within the family change as one person becomes the focus of everyone's efforts and attention. Her mother's illness, and her father's response to it, will affect this little girl as she grows up. Will the early intervention she has had give her the foundation to develop appropriate learning and coping skills in an obviously difficult household? Scientists today are saying that it can.

How Environment Affects IQ

After birth, the brain develops no new neurons. Instead, it forms and breaks connections (synapses) between them at a rapid rate. For the first 8 months, more connections are formed than are broken, but after the first year, there is more pruning—discarding of infrequently used synapses—as the brain reorganizes. Only those synapses that have been called into frequent use survive. Researchers and clinicians agree that social and sensory experience is necessary to wire brain circuitry. The more a synapse is "turned on," the stronger it will become. As the brain develops into maturity, children are able to best use those connections that are activated early, but the brain will re-wire itself throughout life. Therefore, even though the brain has hard-wired itself toward particular habits of thought and behavior by age 3, unless there is chromosomal damage, continuing growth and education (planned, purposeful experiences) can affect personality beyond that age (Kotulak, 1996).

Experience, particularly early experience, also seems to have a profound effect on intelligence—so much so that it is nearly impossible to determine at an early age exactly how functional children affected by Down syndrome and other conditions will become. This is also why there is a lingering debate about whether intellectual capacity is influenced most by nature or by nurture.

One of the earliest (and initially one of the most controversial) studies to demonstrate the power of enrichment experiences on mental development occurred at Glenwood State School for the mentally and physically handicapped in Glenwood, Iowa, in the early 1930s. Twenty-five children from a nearby orphanage were selected to participate in the program. Thirteen toddlers with an average age of 19 months were transferred to the school. There, each baby was given to an individual woman who was mentally handicapped to be cared for. The women gave their young charges lots of attention and affection, stimulated their curiosity, and encouraged them to communicate. The other 12 children remained at the orphanage. The average IQ of the toddlers taken to Glenwood School was 64; the average IQ of those who remained in the orphanage was 87 (Skeels, Updegraff, Wellman, & Williams, 1938).

An 18-month follow-up study showed an average increase of 29 IQ points for the 13 children who had been transferred to the Glenwood School. When the children were re-tested two and a half years later, the 11 who had since been adopted showed an even higher average IQ of 101, and the 12 children who had stayed at the orphanage had lost ground and now had an average IQ of 66 (Skeels et al., 1938).

The idea that IQ is not static did not catch on nationally until 1948, when a study at the University of California at Berkley uncovered new evidence that the intelligent quotient is flexible and can be altered by environment. Berkeley researchers followed 248 urban children from the ages of 18 months to 21 years. During that time period, 60 percent gained at least 15 points in IQ. The other 40 percent made insignificant gains, remained at the same level, or lost ground. Researchers noted that rises in a child's IQ correlated with parents' education level and socioeconomic status, suggesting that external factors impacted gains in IQ (Hawes, 1999).

Those results have never been replicated, but other studies have indeed shown that IQ is enhanced in young children during, or immediately following, enriched education; however, the data qualified that conclusion with evidence that the gains were not permanent if the enrichment occurred after age 3 (Barnett, 2002).

In their work *The Bell Curve: Intelligence and Class Structure in American Life*, published in 1994, Richard Herrnstein and Charles Murray wrote that the data of psychometricians they had studied indicated that hereditary (unalterable) IQ was somewhere between 40 and 80 percent. But their book drew the ire of many of their colleagues because the authors also endorsed social Darwinism—the idea that some races were inherently more intelligent than others—and helped push IQ credibility down.

And theories of gains in intelligence did not necessarily dispute the *g*-factor idea—the general belief that after all is said and done, intelligence is still ultimately stable over time.

Since 2001, however, a new theory has been evolving that postulates that genes and environmental stimuli interact on one another with calculable mathematical precision to increase the intelligence quotient. In other words, they work together predictably. William T. Dickens of The Brookings Institution in Washington, DC, and James R. Flynn of the department of political studies, Universty of Otago, Dunedin, New Zealand, are behind the new vision, which they say "resolves" the dispute over IQ (Dickens & Flynn, 2001).

Not everyone in the scientific community will be convinced, of course, but there is less and less doubt as time goes by that experience acts strongly on developing intelligence.

Emotional Development

It is undisputed that intellectual development cannot go beyond genetic capacity, but early experiences seem to alter the way genes are expressed in the developing brain (Kotulak, 1996). Parents who are pre-occupied with surviving—keeping the family fed, clothed, and sheltered—often do not have the time or resources to interact with their children. As a therapist, you can show the family how to best use the time they have with their children, such as stimulating mental and physical development through ordinary daily activities like getting dressed, doing household chores, and eating meals.

Socio-emotional experiences may outweigh intellectual stimulation in the long-term effect on a child's developing brain (Goleman, 1995). Emotions are produced and controlled by the limbic system, which includes brain structures such as the amygdala, hippocampus, thalamus, and hypothalamus, among others, but almost every part of the brain aids in the expression or inhibition of feelings. If negative concepts are deeply ingrained, or if emotional trauma has occurred, a child's emotional maturation process can come to a standstill or even regress. Suppressing or repressing emotional trauma drives individuals into self-destructive lives, leaving them subconsciously bent on avoiding the unpleasant feelings of anxiety, anger, and depression. As adults, they often learn to self-medicate with drugs or other "anesthetizing" experiences that blot out the pain. We all know of highly intelligent and otherwise successful adults who can barely function as spouses or parents because they seem to be stuck in a particular stage of emotional immaturity. Such people may be unable to take responsibility, to consider the feelings or circumstances of others, or to act with courage when it is necessary.

Emotional problems are not always diagnosable as mental illnesses (there are many shades of gray in what we call mental "health"), but they lower self-worth and impede relationships with others. Physical trauma to the brain sometimes causes psychosocial or emotional problems. People with brain injuries often lose inhibitions, act impulsively, and have difficulty behaving appropriately in social situations. They have to be taught new habits of behavior that will, in turn, re-wire parts of the brain that will take over the functions from the damaged areas of the brain.

Particular kinds of illnesses or disabilities may also have concurrent psychosocial manifestations. For example, children with asthma may develop an inordinate fear of any activity that might trigger an attack. Children whose disabilities are immediately apparent may become shy and withdrawn or act out with aggressive behavior.

Psychosocial Intervention

It is thought that as many as 20 percent of American children may be suffering from a mental illness at any given time (U.S. Department of Health and Human Services, 1999). Because the number of affected children is so high, every EI therapist needs to consider the possible mental health issues in the population he or she is treating. Occupational therapists are not psychologists and should not attempt to be, but they can learn and use basic skills in psychology to understand what they are observing in children and within families. This may mean taking continuing education courses in various aspects of child and adult psychology. Having psychologists or social workers on the team is essential to best practice in EI. Agencies should work together to make sure mental health intervention is available, and these professionals should work in concert with rehabilitation professionals when evaluating needs and planning treatment.

Psychosocial occupational therapy in EI is done within the regular treatment program when the child or parents are resistant to treatment or are not meeting the goals they should be able to meet. Such intervention usually is geared toward motivation, ego support, and alleviation of depression. You do not need to add treatment time to do this. Though any number of physical activities may be used to affect psychosocial outcomes (e.g., drawing, music, toys, games, anything that connects the individual to his emotions), the therapist is the main therapeutic tool. As the Justin's case study illustrates, both parents and children may need to be taught to recognize that certain behaviors reflect their emotional states.

Justin, a short, wiry child was 37 months old when his EI occupational therapy program started. He had been evaluated at 32 months, but his treatment was delayed when his parents separated shortly thereafter. Justin's mother moved him and his 10-month-old sister to her parents' house in a different town.

Justin was delayed in speech and demonstrated a 33-percent delay in fine-motor skills. His cognitive, gross-motor, and sensory abilities were all intact. Justin's mom worked nights, and she believed that her work schedule, the care needed by his infant sister, and the continual difficulties with her husband, had caused Justin's delays. The boy's father was stopping by every other day, but Justin missed having him around. I could see the boy fighting back tears at the mention of his father. As his mom was talking, he suddenly slipped away from her side. He ran to the bay window, reached up above his head and scrambled onto the shelf in a split second. "He's looking for his Dad," she said.

I put several small silk bags on the coffee table and asked him if he would like to see what was inside them. I have used these small make-up bags for many years. They are brightly colored and shaped like envelopes with 3-inch zippers and a snap. I fill them with polished stones; flat, painted wooden fruits and vegetables; miniature animals; found objects (e.g., screws, washers, paper clips, etc.); a few crayons; and small bottles or packs of aromatic herbs. Children love them even before they are old enough to open the bags. Justin was no different. He came over, picked up, felt, and shook each one and chose the one with the stones. His babbling sounded like thrilled language, but no words were distinguishable.

He opened the bag easily and took the stones out one at a time and put them on the table. For each one I named the color. Then I asked him to put them back into the bag by color. He knew colors. He had good manipulative skills but poor graphomotor skills. His mother said she had not played with him using crayons or markers. He began to cry when I gave him a crayon and piece of paper. It seemed clear to me that his fine-motor delay was due to lack of exposure to activities, and that he was as upset about his family situation as his mother. I decided to enhance his fine-motor skills and his self-esteem through creative play.

We played with the contents of the silk bags. He lined up stones for the wooden animals to jump. He made small towers by stacking dominoes with flat wooden pieces and blew them over. I bought more plastic animals so there were large (mommy or daddy) ones and smaller (baby) ones. We made corrals for the different animals so we had families. He learned to make all the animal noises—loud for the bigger animals and very soft for the small ones. I would tell him how much the parents loved their babies. We spent more than six weeks with the animals. He would carefully take them out and put them away at the end. His mom was present during all the sessions. She easily incorporated more cuddle time with him when she saw his response to the animals. I suggested she also verbally reassure him that his father loved him even if he was not there all the time. After Justin grew calmer, I re-introduced crayons and paper. He tentatively began to scribble with different colors and learned to draw vertical and horizontal lines.

(continued)

Late spring came, and we started going outside. He loved to pick dandelions and drop stones into street drains; he loved hearing the stones ping into the water. He was receiving speech therapy twice a week, and he wanted to learn the names of things. His mom was amused that one of his early words was "sewer." On a hill in his own yard, I taught him to roll like a log, turn summersaults, do long jumps, and hop on either foot. He could hop up and down the steep hill.

His grandmother participated in a number of sessions and began to encourage his coloring when I was not there. He learned to hold crayons in a tripod grasp and would scribble papers full of four or five colors and put them on the refrigerator door with magnets. His attention span increased, and his affect became mostly smiles and grins. During his last month of therapy I pushed him to learn to draw shapes. He liked drawing circles but put down his crayon, refusing to try squares or triangles. We both became frustrated, as did his grandmother.

The last session came, and I decided not to push the graphomotor skills, because I knew he would learn these in preschool. Instead, we played with stones and dominoes. Then I gave him a one-inch plastic baby he had not seen before. His eyes lit up when I told him I was going to leave it with him to take care of. Cradling it in his hand, he ran into the kitchen and got a paper napkin. He very carefully swaddled the baby in the soft napkin, held it to his chest and said, "I will take care of you. You will be okay." Then he took my hand and led me to his bedroom. He put the baby doll beside his pillow and carefully tucked it in.

We came back out to the living room, and Justin asked for the crayons. He drew a circle, a square, and a triangle, then turned and hugged me!

Play should be a safe way for children to learn about life. In Justin's case, the tiny toy baby that the therapist gave him put Justin in a "daddy" role. Doing that let him feel the importance of caring for a baby, so that he might understand how his own father felt about him. The act of caring for something tiny allowed him to feel strong and important.

Teaching Self-Control

As children grow up, they need to accept, respect, and express their feelings, but they must learn that they can control their actions even when their emotions are running high. Feelings are prime motivators. Self-worth, optimism, and faith move people forward. Fear, anxiety, self-doubt, and anger often hold them back or keep them mired in unproductive lifestyles.

Before children develop self-control, they depend on external controls to inhibit them. The environment (e.g., a gate across the stairway and caregivers saying "no") makes it more difficult for a child to act on impulse. As children obey their caregivers, they condition themselves toward internal impulse control. Self-control becomes a habit that in turn helps the brain's inhibitory processes mature.

Children learn physical and emotional self-control at the same time. Each milestone in physical self-control can foster emotional self-control, and vice versa. Some parents worry that making a fuss about toilet training will be stressful, or will cause the child to repress or be ashamed of bodily functions. However, it is more likely that a child who is encouraged to use the potty when he or she begins to demonstrate a regular schedule (and may be rewarded with pull-up pants for using it) will feel more competent and content. He or she will be less frustrated and less apt to throw temper tantrums over little things.

For a child's balanced emotional development, it is important for parents and therapists to encourage children to recognize and appropriately express feelings of love, joy, sadness, surprise, fear, anger, and shame by speaking, drawing, coloring, singing, acting, or dancing in a secure environment that allows them to feel that you will not let them lose control entirely. Self-control, which results from discipline, teaches children that they have power over themselves. Their feelings need not rule them.

Fostering Imagination

Imagination—it is one of your most potent psychosocial tools. Imagination is more than just a means of entertainment; it is part of the brain's growth process. Brain activity is divided into two categories, each handled by different sides of the brain. The left brain, which normally operates most often in adults, controls rational thought, verbalization, and other processes connected to physical reality. The right brain controls synthetic, holistic, intuitive perception, and information processing. It is the seat of creativity. In the very young, free play develops the right side of the brain. Free play should be unfettered play. Toys that "do everything for you" take imagination out of the equation. Though some educational toys promise to increase cognitive development, artistic development and problem-solving skills usually take a back seat. One preschool girl who had all the latest toys at home hardly ever played with them, but when she went to her grandmother's house, where there were only a few toys, she spent hours building towers, gardens, and houses with plain wooden blocks and plastic animals and plants.

The trick to encouraging imagination in children is to give them toys that are symbolic of life: people, animals, cars and trucks, things to build with, old clothes to dress up in, and simple household items they can turn into other toys. Being read to from an early age also helps a child learn to imagine different creatures, places, people, and circumstances, and to imagine what is possible as well as what exists now. Imagination, fired by desire and molded by realistic constructs, is what has brought forth most of the great inventions of history. It can also be especially powerful in helping traumatized children heal.

Combating Overstimulation

As important as stimulation is to the mind-growing process, too much of it can be disabling. Picture yourself in a foreign land where people look very different from you; you do not know the language, and the everyday items they use are unfamiliar. This is roughly the situation of an infant or very young child. Now imagine that you are at a carnival in this place, where everything new is going on at once. Your first impulse might be to escape the scene and go find a place where you can quietly organize your thoughts.

The younger the infant you see in EI, especially if he or she was born prematurely, the more likely he or she is to be dealing with issues related to overstimulation. In fact, parents tend to overburden their young children with too many toy attractions, too many bright colors, and too many people. In such homes, you may find yourself suggesting some environmental modification—using household items as playthings, putting out only a few toys at a time, and quieting the room with appropriate music. At all ages, the brain needs time to organize information in order to make sense of it. Literally everything a newborn sees, smells, tastes, or touches is foreign. The developing brain becomes easily overwhelmed and babies must be protected from overstimulation, particularly premature babies.

Because babies cannot talk, they have to show you when they are uncomfortable. Crying is only one of their methods of communication. Babies will also look away from something that is too much for them to process. Even seeing more than one face at a time or a face that is showing too much feeling can become overwhelming for an infant (Peterson-DeGoff, 2003). Overstimulated babies may close their eyes and try to sleep, or stick out their tongues and then yawn. If the baby begins to arch his or her back and tries to move away or begins to get cranky, the environment is probably too stimulating. Caregivers should modulate stimulation to make it less overwhelming.

Many schools of infant and child education recommend natural media as the best growing tools. They believe most of today's commercially sold "educational" toys have too many bells and whistles.

Rudolph Steiner (1861–1925), founded the Waldorf Schools, known for their open-ended approach to education. Waldorf Schools developed a theory which proposes that children pay different types of attention to different objects. According to the Waldorf philosophy, when a child focuses on an object, the neural pathways that he or she will need for later use in concentration are developed. In order to best develop these neural pathways, Waldorf encourages exposing children to objects or activities that foster "deep attentiveness, long, curious staring and wondering…pastel colors; a feather on a string, spinning in the breeze; a fish tank to watch; curtains blowing; lying under a tree; a candle flame…."(Peterson-DeGoff, 2003). Given the near epidemic of attention-deficit disorders among children today, a theory which suggests a way to approach development of concentration bears some consideration.

THE 12 THEORIES OF LEARNING

Early intervention is meant to prepare children for school readiness by identifying early any barriers that are likely to impede their success, and intervening to bring children up to the skill standards of their age group. Each person learns in his or her own way; however, and you will need different approaches for different children. Personality and temperament make them all unique. Some are eager to try new things; others are resistant. Some "get it" quickly; others take more time. Toys that fascinate one kid can leave another looking around the room in boredom.

What turns the key to your young client's mind?

Listed below are 12 theories of learning that each take slightly different slants on the process. See which ones you agree with most.

(continued)

1. Constructivism

Constructivism is a philosophy of learning founded on the premise that, by reflecting on our experiences, we construct our own understanding of the world we live in. Each of us generates our own "rules" and "mental models," which we use to make sense of our experiences. Learning, therefore, is simply the process of adjusting our mental models to accommodate new experiences. *Learning is a search for meaning.*

2. Behaviorism

Behavior theorists define learning as nothing more than the acquisition of new behavior. Experiments by behaviorists identify conditioning as a universal learning process. There are two different types of conditioning, each yielding a different behavioral pattern: Classical conditioning is what Pavlov sees when he observes that dogs salivate when they eat or even see food. Essentially, animals and people are biologically "wired" so that a certain stimulus will produce a specific response. Behavioral or operant conditioning occurs when a response to a stimulus is reinforced. If a reward or reinforcement follows the response to a stimulus, then the response becomes more probable in the future.

3. Piaget's Model

Swiss biologist and psychologist Jean Piaget (1896–1980) is renowned for constructing a highly influential model of child development and learning. Piaget's theory is based on the idea that the developing child builds cognitive structures. He identifies four developmental stages and the processes by which children progress through them. Two of them apply to children in early intervention: the sensorimotor stage (birth–2 years old), when the child, through physical interaction with his or her environment, builds a set of concepts about reality and how it works; and the preoperational stage (ages 2–7), when the child is not yet able to conceptualize abstractly and needs concrete physical situations.

4. Neuroscience

Neuroscience studies the human nervous system, the brain, and the biological basis of consciousness, perception, memory, and learning. It links our observations about cognitive behavior with the actual physical processes that support such behavior. This theory is still young and is undergoing rapid, controversial development.

5. Brain-Based Learning

This learning theory also is based on the structure and function of the brain. As long as the brain is not prohibited from fulfilling its normal processes, learning will occur.

People often say that everyone can learn. Yet the reality is that everyone does learn. Every person is born with a brain that functions as an immensely powerful processor. Traditional schooling, however, often inhibits learning by discouraging, ignoring, or punishing the brain's natural learning processes.

(continued)

6. Learning Styles

This approach to learning emphasizes the fact that individuals perceive and process information in very different ways. The learning styles theory implies that how much individuals learn has more to do with whether the educational experience is geared toward their particular style of learning than whether or not they are "smart." In fact, educators should not ask, "Is this student smart?" but rather "How is this student smart?"

7. Multiple Intelligences

Psychologist Howard Gardner suggests there are at least seven ways that people have of perceiving and understanding the world. Gardner labels each of these ways a distinct "intelligence"—in other words, a set of skills allowing individuals to find and resolve genuine problems they face.

While Gardner suggests his list of intelligences may not be exhaustive, he identifies the following seven:

- **Verbal-Linguistic**—The ability to use words and language.

- **Logical-Mathematical**—The capacity for inductive and deductive thinking and reasoning, as well as the use of numbers and the recognition of abstract patterns.

- **Visual-Spatial**—The ability to visualize objects and spatial dimensions, and create internal images and pictures.

- **Body-Kinesthetic**—The wisdom of the body and the ability to control physical motion.

- **Musical-Rhythmic**—The ability to recognize tonal patterns and sounds, as well as a sensitivity to rhythms and beats.

- **Interpersonal**—The capacity for person-to-person communications and relationships.

- **Intrapersonal**—The spiritual, inner states of being, self-reflection, and awareness.

8. Right Brain versus Left Brain

This theory of the structure and functions of the mind suggests that the two different sides of the brain control two different "modes" of thinking. It also suggests that each of us prefers one mode over the other.

9. Communities of Practice

This approach views learning as an act of membership in a "community of practice." The theory seeks to understand both the structure of communities and how learning occurs in them.

(continued)

10. Control Theory

This theory of motivation proposed by William Glasser contends that behavior is never caused by a response to an outside stimulus. Instead, the control theory states that behavior is inspired by what a person *wants* most at any given time: survival, love, power, freedom, or any other basic human need. *Glasser attests that all living creatures "control" their behavior to maximize their need satisfaction. According to Glasser, if students are not motivated to do their schoolwork, it's because they view schoolwork as irrelevant to their basic human needs.*

11. Observational Learning

Observational learning, also called social learning theory, occurs when an observer's behavior changes after viewing the behavior of a model. An observer's behavior can be affected by the positive or negative consequences—called vicarious reinforcement or vicarious punishment—of a model's behavior. The observer will imitate the model's behavior if the model possesses characteristics—things such as talent, intelligence, power, good looks, or popularity—that the observer finds attractive or desirable.

12. Vygotsky and Social Cognition

The social cognition learning model asserts that culture is the prime determinant of individual development. Humans are the only species to have created culture, and every human child develops in the context of a culture. Therefore, a child's learning development is affected in ways large and small by the culture—including the culture of family environment—in which he or she is enmeshed.

_____

Published by Funderstanding, Livingston, NJ. Content by On Purpose Assoc. *Reprinted with permission.*

Nutrition's Role in Behavior

There is good evidence to support the old truism that you are what you eat. Your young clients will show you how this works very quickly, as their behavior is likely to be influenced by their diets.

Many children today begin consuming sugary cereals and drinks as soon as they can physically handle spoons and cups. Pasta is introduced early as a finger food and pancakes, doughnuts, pizza, fruits, and fruit juices are all typical toddler fare. The result is that refined sugars and simple carbohydrates compose an inordinate amount of the diet of most young children.

Attention deficit disorders are being linked to diet and digestive processes and also to lack of sleep. Though ADD and ADHD are not usually diagnosed until a child is 6 or 7, nutritional habits in toddlerhood can promote these problems or help arrest them. Refined sugars and de-fibered starches are metabolized quickly and push the blood sugar up and down like a roller coaster as insulin pours in to help the cells process those ingredients. Insulin "dumps" after high-carbohydrate meals drop blood sugar quickly, and interfere with the brain's ability to keep its fuel at constant levels. This may be particularly harmful to a young child, whose brain is still developing. In an effort to make up for what they are not getting (or getting too much of), body systems rebalance. To "wake themselves up," so to speak, children with attention deficit disorders move. They keep up a steady pace of running, climbing, fidgeting, tapping, changing positions, talking, and focusing on different things. This diverts them from concentrating, except for short periods of time. Higher protein diets with complex carbohydrates (whole grains) have been found to help reduce the effects of ADD or ADHD in many cases (Amen, 2001).

What role diet and metabolism play in the autism spectrum is not known, but there is some evidence that glutens (from wheat) and caseins (from dairy products) are involved in aspects of some forms of autism. The speculation, not very widely agreed upon at this point, is that these products, which produce natural opioids, somehow interfere with chemical transmission in the brain (Shattock, 1995). Researchers know that brain chemistry involves the transmission of messages from neuron to neuron via neurotransmitters such as serotonin, norepinephrin, and other chemicals that "bounce" back and forth between the synapses of nerves the way a baseball does between the pitcher and catcher. Receptors ("gloves") on the "players" receive and decode the messages.

The Development of Self-Concept

Children and adults learn to judge their worth by what they can do, as seen through the responses of other people (e.g., Are Mom and Dad impressed with me? Or are they indifferent? Then I must not have done it well enough.). The development of self is the development of ego, the "I am" of the mind. In infancy, the sense of self is highly fluid. Babies associate everything they sense with themselves—there are no boundaries between "you" and "me." As children grow, they learn that they exist independently from others. The child is not Mommy, Daddy, or siblings. The child's toys belong to him but they are not part of him. He will not cease to exist if someone takes them out of sight.

Infants and young children mirror what they see their parents and siblings doing. They imitate other people's behavior while looking back to see if their parents are watching. Children interpret who they are and how valuable they are by the visual, auditory, and tactile responses they receive from others in the home. This feedback plays upon genetic predispositions, but the quality of these encounters will reflect in the roles a child will play and the relationships he or she will have with other people as the child grows up.

Self-Concept and the Child With Disabilities

An infant with disabilities greatly impacts the living environment because the child needs more of the parents' attention and time than other children in the family. Both parents and even the siblings organize their lives around the infant. One or both parents may have to stop working to care for the child. In the beginning there may be constant monitoring of the newborn's vital signs, and it may take all day to get enough food into the baby. Medical service personnel may disrupt the routine even more by making multiple visits. Siblings may be beset with conflicting feelings—worry about the survival of their new brother or sister mixed with resentment and jealousy that so much has been taken from them for his or her sake.

The mother's emotional attitude may be permanently changed. She may overprotect the child. She may secretly resent the child and adopt a passive-aggressive attitude toward him or her. She may blame herself for the baby's disability and try to "make up" for it. As long as the child is disabled, she will spend more of her energy on him or her, coaching the child toward as much independence as he or she can handle.

Because of such "circling of the wagons," most very young children with disabilities get used to being the center of attention. They may expect other people to help them do things they could do for themselves if they tried. They have to concentrate more mental and physical effort on doing things other children can do easily, and they may have a harder time stepping back from themselves to see the big picture. It is important to help them understand that they are special not because they need special attention, but because, just like their non-disabled peers, they have their own inborn talents and gifts of skill to be developed. One of the most important developmental stages all people need to transit is to see outside themselves. For people with disabilities, making that transit is harder, but it is well worth the effort, for it will become the key to reciprocal, satisfying relationships with others in their lives (Hwang, 1997).

Parents are the key to this transition in self concept, and it is important that they recover from the initial shock of their situation. Every family is different. Some seem to have boundless energy to meet these new challenges. They become proactive advocates immediately. Other families get caught in one or another of the aspects of the problem and cannot seem to gain momentum. Still other families are overwhelmed by the circumstances and need professional help. Your job is to assess the situation in the home, determine what needs are to be met, and help parents find the resources they need. This is family-based intervention.

FOOD FOR THOUGHT

- What roles do you believe "nature" and "nurture" play in child development?
- Justin's therapist used toys to help him understand what families are. How did she use role play to help him connect to his own feelings? Why did it work?
- Of the 12 theories of learning, which two seem the most valid to you? How would you use them in teaching a young child?

Development in Motion

5

MAGGIE'S STORY

Maggie was 34 months old and absolutely adorable. She had been born with Erb's palsy, a birth injury to the brachial plexus that had permanently affected her arm. Maggie had sensation but less than 30 percent motion in her shoulder, elbow, and wrist. Her entire hand was non-functional, with the exception of gross motor control over her thumb and one finger. Prior therapy had focused entirely on her arm and hand, and her mother had been taught how to range the extremity and do proprioceptive neuromuscular facilitation (PNF) to stimulate the nerves and muscles. The arm had neither atrophied nor contracted, and her disability was not apparent.

The problem now was Maggie's behavior. In the past few months Maggie had become impossible according to her mother. She was uncooperative and had frequent temper tantrums, throwing her toys or anything in reach. She had become a very fussy eater and had to be bribed to eat by the promise of a spoonful of rice pudding after each bite. Each night she woke up and crawled into her parents' bed, screaming at the top of her lungs if either of them tried to move her. She had made no attempt to learn to dress herself, although her one fully functional arm made her physically capable of putting on simple clothing. The mother had not begun toilet training because it upset Maggie. As her mother and I talked, Maggie took sips from a baby bottle—she was not weaned, either.

Maggie's mother was a college graduate, a dancer, and a free-spirited woman who believed in letting things happen "naturally." She believed developmental milestones were artificially and arbitrarily assigned. She did not want guidance to help Maggie meet milestones; she wanted to learn when Maggie would outgrow this "phase." I told her mother that Maggie would learn self-control by learning first that she could control her own body. I explained that milestones are flexible points that reflect a child's readiness, both physically and psychologically, to learn higher-level tasks. They allow the child to embrace more of the surrounding world by training the body. In a way, I compared it to the mother learning a new, more complicated dance move that allowed her more freedom in dance.

First, we made a plan to wean Maggie by offering her fruit juice in a small glass with a wide stem so she could easily hold it in one hand. She was allowed to eat at the table in a booster seat for the first time. It took less than a week for Maggie to give up the bottle. She really had been ready and waiting.

Toilet training was a bit harder. Fortunately, it was summer and the family had a large, fenced-in yard. Using an old fashioned method, we let Maggie play outside without her diapers and with a potty chair nearby. Maggie's mother laughed out loud when she described the look on Maggie's face when she wet herself. "That's why grown ups use toilets–so we don't get wet," her mother explained. Maggie started using the potty chair and wearing her Tinker Bell panties.

As Maggie began to feel more grown-up, her tantrums diminished and she spontaneously began to try to dress herself. Her mother was thrilled, and with some instruction began to encourage higher level one-handed activities. Maggie will always have only one fully functioning hand, and it needs to become highly skilled to do the work of both. Maggie's mother came to realize that developmental milestones played an important role in guiding Maggie to maturity.

Evolving Thought in Child Development

Child development gets a lot of press these days, and "milestones" is a word many parents already know. You might think that the focus on milestones is a highly modern approach to rearing children, but it has been around for almost 100 years. Arnold Gesell, MD, PhD, opened the Yale Clinic of Child Development in a small room at the New Haven Dispensary in 1911. Known as the father of child development in the United States, he was both a physician and a psychologist. In the 1920s he used cinema analysis to document the milestone development of children from infancy through adolescence. His most famous book, *An Atlas of Infant Behavior*, contains 3,200 action photographs of babies and children as they grow up (Yale Child Study Center, 2003).

Dr. Benjamin Spock, who died in 1998, wrote the bestselling child care book of all time, *The Common Sense Book of Baby and Child Care*, first published in 1946. He "oversaw" the rearing of the entire baby-boom generation and of their children. Spock was a trained psychotherapist as well as a physician, and he revolutionized general public thought about the parent-child relationship, making it clear that unconditional love and affection were the backbone of that bond and the prime movers in growing healthy children.

In 1945, Columbia University medical graduate T. Berry Brazelton began his residency at Massachusetts General Hospital in Boston, where he took training in child psychiatry at Boston Children's Hospital. He went on to become one of the most famous child development specialists in the country. In 1972 he established the child development unit in pediatrics training and research at Boston's Children's Hospital. His Neonatal Behavioral Assessment Scale (NBAS), first published in 1973, and most recently revised in 1995, is now known as "The Brazelton," and is used worldwide to assess the physical, neurological, and emotional responses of newborns as well as their individual differences.

In 2001, the authors retooled the scale to a shorter form that clinicians could use in hospitals or homes, and called it the Clinical Neonatal Behavioral Assessment Scale (CLNBAS) but did not republish it.

The scale, in either form, is commonly known as "The Brazelton." It identifies 28 behavioral and 18 reflex items designed to test the infant's physiological, motor, and social capacities over a two-month period.

In 2005, the Brazelton Institute changed the name of its clinical assessment to the Newborn Behavioral Observation System (NBO), grouping its items into observation groups designed to strengthen the relationship among parents, children, and clinicians. The new tool is expected to publish in 2006.

The NBO system helps physicians and parents create a profile of the baby that will not only detect abnormalities but also try to capture the baby's individuality by creating an overview of his or her strengths from the details. This tool also has been lauded for helping build parent-child relationships and for teaching parents their baby's communication cues to share with physicians so they can all work together to help the baby grow.

Stages of Early Childhood Development

Development begins immediately after birth, when newborns begin working to control three bodily systems. The first system, the autonomic nervous system (ANS), regulates breathing and body temperature. At birth even slight changes in temperature or environment can startle an infant or make the skin change color. Once the ANS is under control, infants try to control their motor responses. Holding or swaddling newborns helps them stop random movements and get muscles working voluntarily. State-of-consciousness, or arousal control, is next on the agenda. Arousal is a continuum that runs from quiet sleep to full cry. The baby needs to transition along this continuum in order to be able to process and respond to stimuli in the environment. Some babies easily tune out light and noises and sleep through them. Others are much more aware of changes and are easily awakened. Only after achieving these three tasks can infants finally start to really take notice of the world around them (Brazelton & Nugent, 1995).

Birth to 8 Months

Zero to Three, a nonprofit organization focused on early childhood development, has compiled one of the most parent-friendly child development charts on the Internet called "Developmental Milestones: How I Grow In Your Care." It features a developmental timeline divided into three parts: young infants (birth to 8 months), explorers (8 to 18 months), and toddlers and two-year olds (18 months through 2 years). You can find it at: http://www.zerotothree.org/dev_miles.html. We will paraphrase the timeline and use some of its specific language to illustrate what an infant or toddler is experiencing at any given age. It is important to remember that milestones are only guidelines. Normal development is a continuum along which an infant or toddler may move forward or backward over a period of time—but he or she should move backward only temporarily.

In the first 8 months, infants examine and use their bodies and learn that they can trust their parents to come when they are needed, and hold or comfort them if necessary. Sucking on something can comfort infants until their parents arrive. Eventually, babies discover they can make things happen autonomously by shaking a rattle or kicking a mobile.

Motor skills come one at a time. Newborns look for something to put in their mouths, and turn their heads to breathe if the nose or mouth is blocked. Bright lights make infants squint or turn away. In a few months infants will be able to hold something, let it go, and pick it up again, and move an object from one hand to the other. This is the beginning of purposeful movement, and it changes the way infants use their muscles.

Infants are also learning about feelings. When infants show feelings, they want their parents to understand and help control them when they become overwhelming. By the end of this period, as egos bud, infants begin to realize that they are autonomous. The parents are separate from the child. Hide-and-seek and peek-a-boo teach babies that if someone "disappears," he will come back, and the child can do the same.

Infants in this stage will sometimes cry if a stranger holds or even looks at them. They are fearful of unknown people until someone they trust shows them that they are all right. One 8-month-old girl cried at the sight of her grandmother, who had come to visit from another state, until the girl's 4-year-old brother rushed into the grandmother's arms. Then the baby looked surprised, smiled, and held out her own arms. Family members are much more interesting to an 8-month-old than toys, because the baby can "talk" to them and they will respond. Babies this age will begin to hold "conversations" with their families with coos, babbles, gurgles, "mamas," and "dadas."

Months 8–18

Beginning at about 8 months, infants become recognizable people. From crawling to cruising to walking to running, they are constantly on the move. They may want to do more than they can handle, and may resist parents' efforts to slow them down. Two-way communication is important now. Infants know when their parents are talking at them instead of to them. They lose respect for themselves when they feel ignored or "patronized." They like to be invited to help, and praise buoys their spirit. They feel confident when their parents let them try new things.

The "terrible twos" are not so terrible, and they usually start before age 2. Ego development now reaches a stage where children learn they are separate beings and realize they must behave as individuals. This identity quest sets up a conflict of wills between parent and child that will continue to play itself out as parents learn to feel comfortable letting infants become children who can express their own wills. Learning how to understand and handle this is an important step for parents and children.

Somewhere around 18 months, children start saying "no!" to everything. They will pull people where they want them to be, or push them off their favorite chair. They may begin to fight for their "territory" (e.g., toys, a favorite person's lap, etc.). They begin to use "me," "I," and "mine." When they are angry they may hit, push, or even bite to prevail. They will also shriek with joy and run into their parents' arms to give them a hug. They will want them to watch their every move. They may also try to stop their parents from leaving the house—it frightens young children when those important to them are gone. However, by this time, children are well on their way to learning that when people leave, they also return. A consistent daily schedule helps children understand and predict what will happen.

By 18 months, children have favorite toys and foods, and like to choose what to wear. They make silly faces and noises with other children and may pretend to play house, ride a train, or talk on the phone. They are not likely to share without prompting, but can be taught to take turns. They will imitate what their parents do, such as walking the dog on a leash or pushing the vacuum cleaner around. If the ball goes behind the sofa, they may look for it. Tool use begins at about 18 months, and children may use one object to try to manipulate another.

By 18 months old, children will mark things with crayons using a prehensile grip, may stack or line up blocks, can finger-feed, use a spoon, and drink from a cup. They can sit in a chair, help to dress themselves, walk backwards a few steps, and try to climb stairs on all fours. They will create babble sentences and may say two or three words. They will look their parents in the eye to get their attention and point to interesting pictures and objects, wanting to hear about them. They will turn their attention to objects the family members talk about.

18 Months–3 Years

By the age of 2, most children can say from three to ten words, although parents may not understand them. Two-year-olds sometimes feel very powerful because of all the successes they have had. They test their parents in everything, but they want their parents to set clear limits because independence can be scary. They have a sense of belonging to a family and of using "their" language. At this age, children feel safe when the household operates routinely and peacefully. They recognize family pictures hanging on the walls.

By 2–3 years old, children sense things very well. They are sensitive to insults and dislike being called ugly, dumb, or bad. When disciplining, parents should always criticize the act, not the child, and should do so fairly. When praising, they should be honest and emphasize successful parts of the effort. They should avoid praising every small task a child completes. Values and skills are learned through repetition and corrections. Self-control is developing and toilet training helps that happen.

Children at this age now begin to fear imaginary things, like the monster under the bed, the dark, or people in masks or costumes. These children are learning to play with others, to "imagine together," and often mimic the scenes they see at home. They learn how to treat others from the way they see their parents treat people. Both boys and girls often offer sympathy if they see a parent hurting or unhappy. A parent's persistent unhappiness may make a child fearful. Children are aware of who should be present in a particular group, and they like to explore the environment together. Although they understand that they should share, they may still find difficulty with it.

Children who are 2–3 years old can group objects and can find similar toys in a bag, even with their eyes closed. They can kick and throw a ball, stand on one foot, walk upstairs putting one foot on each step, and are beginning to build block towers. They can thread beads with large holes, and draw some shapes, like circles. They may know numbers all the way up to 10. They can dress themselves in simple clothes and can pour milk on their own cereal.

During this stage, children's language may suddenly blossom. Children in the third year may know 200 words in their primary language and sometimes as many in a second language. They can tell you about things that happened in the past, and things that will happen in the future. They may need some time to make themselves understood, and listeners should be patient.

By 3 years old, children like to hear stories read to them and like to "read" the stories back. Sometimes they will join in when their mother or father tells a story. They also like to sing, often have a favorite song, and talk to other children as they act out scenes together. They can understand some symbols, like using a block for a phone.

Debunking Developmental Misconceptions

Although developmental milestones are generally agreed upon by child development experts, research shows that some parents may have unreasonably high expectations of their toddlers' capacity for self-control and reduced awareness of their emotional reactions. What parents believe about their infant influences how they behave toward the infant. When parents' expectations do not correspond with actual child development, parents may inappropriately discipline a child when they should be guiding the child.

Zero to Three conducted a national survey ("What Grown-Ups Understand About Child Development: A National Benchmark Survey," 2000) among parents who had children from newborn to 6 years of age. The study found that misconceptions about child development were common.

- 55 percent of parents believed an infant must be 3 months of age or older to sense the mood of the parent. Fathers and adults who plan to be future parents most often believe the infant must be a year or older. In reality, infants as young as a month old can be affected by parents' moods, and there is some evidence that even fetuses can be affected by their mothers' moods (Fassler & Dumas, 1997).

- 51 percent of parents believed that a 15-month-old should be able to share toys. In reality, even with help, children are not ready to do that consistently until they are over 2 years old.

- 26 percent of parents believed that a 3-year-old should be able to sit quietly for an hour. While some 3-year-olds might be able to do that, most need to have diversionary toys, or other objects to keep them busy.

- 39 percent of parents (and 46 percent of all adults who participated in the survey) believed that a 1-year-old child who walked up to the TV and tried to turn it on and off repeatedly while the parents were watching was doing it to annoy the parents. (The majority, however, believed it was for attention, or simply because the child wanted to see what happened when the buttons were pressed.) In reality, repetition is a strong characteristic of children this age, who are "growing" their motor systems.

Can You Spoil a Child?

There is still a strong dichotomy of attitudes in the United States about spoiling young children (e.g., teaching them to expect more than they "should" have). The Zero to Three survey showed that fathers, grandparents, and parents with high-school degrees or less had very strong fears about spoiling. Fifty percent of fathers and 63 percent of grandparents polled believed that picking up a three-month-old every time he or she cried would spoil the infant. Child development researchers disagree. They claim, with supporting research, that even six-month-olds are too young to spoil with excessive attention (Commons & Miller, 1998).

All parents have their own ideas when it comes to discipline, but *how* children are corrected may matter more than when they are corrected. Child development experts agree that consistency is the most important aspect of effective discipline, because self-control is a habit-driven skill. In order to help children develop self-control, parents need to learn what their children are truly capable of at any given age. Be aware that misconceptions about child development are common, and be prepared to educate parents about developmental milestones if necessary.

Determining the Causes of Regression

Most children will continue to progress normally through developmental milestones, but some parents may notice that their child suddenly seems to be going backwards—losing skills instead of gaining them. A young child who could walk will suddenly stop walking and start crawling, or one who could talk stops talking and becomes completely uncommunicative or uses unintelligible language. These are rare but serious symptoms that need to be evaluated quickly by the proper medical professionals because certain physical and psychiatric illnesses can cause this kind of regression.

Sometimes children who have been meeting milestones can be temporarily delayed or may even regress when faced with an unusually stressful situation in the home. If a child's regression coincides with a dramatic change in the home environment, such as the birth of another baby, stress may be the cause. In the absence of a medical cause of regression, loving encouragement is usually all these children need to begin progressing in their development again.

FOOD FOR THOUGHT

- How long has child development been under study by medical personnel? Should developmental milestones be used as prognosticators or guidelines in assessing progress and delay?

- Why is the CLNBAS one of the most comprehensive tools to use for developmental assessment? What other tools have you discovered that are good for assessing children's emotional and social development?

- Were you surprised to learn how much parents do not know about children's behavior and development? Why do you think this problem exists, and how will you, as a therapist, help reverse the trend with the families you treat?

- How can you train parents and caregivers to use early intervention options to their fullest potential?

Some Diagnoses in EI: An Outline of Medical Conditions

Children are automatically referred for EI services if they are very premature, have been in neonatal intensive care, or if they have been diagnosed at birth with a specific medical condition or disorder. There are other problems that do not manifest until sometime within the first three years of life, which make vigilance on the part of parents and physicians very important. Diagnostic categories are becoming more complex as researchers try to isolate groupings of symptoms, identify their origins, and create new treatment regimens. Most delays you will see in gross- and fine-motor development are environmentally driven and will resolve with the right treatment. They are not the result of pathology; however, you will also see many highly involved children whose delays are part of medically complex syndromes. Even if there is a medical diagnosis for a child, it may or may not be listed on the Individual Family Service Plan (IFSP). Once a diagnosis has been made and you believe you need to see it, you must have the permission of both the parents and the doctor to get it under new the HIPAA privacy regulations. Even if the parents agree to allow you to have the diagnosis information, the physician is still, by law, allowed to say no. Most doctors are not likely to go that far.

What follows is an alphabetical synopsis of the types of disabilities you might see in EI, their etiology and symptomatology, and their functional prognosis. Dr. Mark L. Batshaw's book *Children With Disabilities, 5th Edition* (2002), is one of the best medical resources available for early intervention.

Chromosomal and Genetic Disorders

Diagnoses: Turner syndrome, Williams syndrome, Klinefelter syndrome, trisomy 13 syndrome, Edwards syndrome, Duchenne muscular dystrophy (DMD), phenylketonuria (PKU; see Developmental Disabilities/Mental Retardation) Down syndrome (see Developmental Disabilities/Mental Retardation), fragile x (see Developmental Disabilities/Mental Retardation), cleft lip/palate (see Hearing and Speech Disorders), neural tube deficits (see Neural Tube Defects), mitochondrial disorders

Etiology: genetic errors that include, among others, trisomy 21, mosaicism, translocation, deletion, inversion and mutations (Batshaw, 2002, pp. 7–13).

Symptoms: The syndromes listed above are usually visible because they involve congenital abnormalities in the facial features, neck, and/or head. They are also associated with myriad medical problems that complicate the conditions. DMD has no such visible signs. Children with the disease develop enlargement of the calves and muscle weakness that worsens as they grow older. In DMD there is no cognitive decline.

Prognoses: Very involved children with many of these disorders will need lifelong care. Some will have shortened life spans. Others (born with fewer abnormalities) may progress, with adaptive equipment and supportive parenting, through the stages of childhood with continued assistance.

Impact on Family Life and Future Education: Parents and siblings of children with any of these disorders will spend much time attempting to bring better quality of life to these children. If children have multiple medical problems, parents' lives can become entwined with treatment regimens. Even if intelligence is normal, adaptations will have to be made for schooling. The child's lifespan may be uncertain. These families also need to prepare for their child's care in the event of their own deaths.

Developmental Disabilities and Mental Retardation

Diagnosis: ADHD (attention deficit hyperactivity disorder)

Etiology: The origin of these fairly new diagnostic categories is still debated. These conditions may manifest alone or as part of certain medical conditions. They are classified as neurobehavioral syndromes in individuals who display inappropriate levels of attention or activity that impairs functioning at home or school because of the inability to achieve or maintain full-focused consciousness (Batshaw, 2002, p. 389). There are varying subtypes of the disorder that often manifest differently in boys and girls. Recently, lack of sleep has been suspected of aggravating these problems. ADHD is not usually diagnosed in the early intervention setting, but symptoms may become visible there. Early testing in vision and hearing may help offset later problems, and consistency in disciplinary approaches may help these children learn self-discipline and self-control. Most children with these syndromes have only slight abnormalities of brain function. The tendency toward ADHD seems to be passed down from one generation to another. Perceptual, as well as nutritional factors (not always easily identified), also can play into this syndrome, which makes it even more difficult to diagnose.

Symptoms: General symptoms in these two disorders include lack of ability to stay on task or to concentrate on one thing. Children with the combined type ADHD may be revved up and always moving, often impulsively. Those with the inattentive type of ADHD tend to be more distracted, or "off in a dream world." They have trouble paying attention to directions, do not remember sequential directions, and often lose things (Batshaw, 2002, pp. 390–391).

Prognosis: The most important predictor of prognosis is the accurate diagnosis of the problem(s) that underlies the behavior. The drug Ritalin®, a stimulant, is widely used to alleviate ADHD symptoms, but its use today is heavily debated among parents, and you are not likely to see it used in children 3 and under. Many families (and some doctors) now do not want to put even school-age youngsters on Ritalin. Some families have had success with diet and nutrition changes and others with behavioral approaches.

Impact on Family Life and Future Education: ADHD wreaks havoc on the family because of behavioral issues. These children are very hard to deal with and try everyone's patience. They have problems in school and with socialization. If a child in EI shows such symptoms, it is important to find out what might be causing them. If no physical or psychological problems can be found, the children may simply not be disciplined appropriately or consistently. Parents need to be taught how to instill in their children the skills they will use to control themselves as they get older. An accurate history of infancy and developmental milestones helps divide behavioral issues from pathology.

Diagnosis: Autistic disorder (see PDD)

Diagnosis: Down syndrome (trisomy 21); (see entry in Chromosomal Disorders)

Etiology: Chromosomal abnormalities account for the three types of Down syndrome, identified visually by Dr. John Langdon Down in 1866. Trisomy 21 is involved in 95 percent of Down syndrome cases; Translocation Down is seen in about 4 percent of cases, and mosaic trisomy in only 1 percent. There is little difference in effect between the first two types, but in mosaic Down syndrome, the trisomic cells are interspersed with normal cells, and these children score up to 30 points higher on IQ tests than the others do (Batshaw, 2002, pp. 307–308).

Symptoms: Mental retardation is present to varying degrees, and there is increased risk of abnormalities in many organs. These children may also have congenital heart disease, ophthalmic disorders, hearing disorders, endocrine abnormalities, celiac disease, dental problems and growth problems. Sensory impairments are common in children with Down syndrome (Batshaw, 2002, pp. 309–313).

Prognosis: The degree of cognitive involvement is paramount in the prognosis. It is important to give higher-functioning Down syndrome children the opportunity to take part in all that they can in order to give them experience in mastering living skills. Some can lead independent but supervised lives by adulthood.

Impact on Family Life and Future Education: Although they take a lot of nurturing, children with Down syndrome are normally good-natured and loving, and they give their parents something in return for the care they get. Some can progress through special education to the point of high school "graduation," but many will stay in special education programs until they reach 21.

Diagnosis: Fragile x syndrome

Etiology: The most frequently diagnosed inherited cause of mental retardation, fragile x syndrome, is an x-linked genetic disorder responsible for one-third of all x-linked causes of mental retardation and 40 percent of x-linked learning disabilities. DNA testing is necessary to diagnose fragile x (Batshaw, 2002, p. 321).

Symptoms: Speech-language delay; marked hyperactivity; self-stimulatory behavior; in girls, excessive shyness. The condition is much more obvious in boys, who may present with large, protruding ears, hyperextensible joints, flat feet, ophthalmic problems, and (not as often) macrocephaly. In girls, these traits are less visible. The girls may have non-language-based learning disabilities and may tend to be shy or withdrawn. In either sex, mental retardation may or may not be present (Batshaw, 2002, pp. 322–323).

Prognosis: Early diagnosis can aid intervention, especially in speech/language pathology, that will help these children get a good start, but many will need lifelong supervision. Lifespan is generally normal for both sexes (Batshaw, 2002, p. 328).

Impact on Family Life and Future Education: Fragile x children require a lot of love and patience. Getting them through to the best adult outcome possible takes almost single-minded attention on the part of parents. Higher functioning girls with fragile x are more likely to be able to live on their own or with minimum supervision, but they face the possibility of acquiring psychiatric disturbances if the gene is fully mutated. Boys' behavior problems and social skills deficits hamper their ability to live independently (Batshaw, 2002, p. 328).

Diagnosis: Fetal alcohol syndrome (FAS); alcohol-related neurodevelopmental disorder (ARND); alcohol-related birth defects

Etiology: Ingested alcohol affects development and function of the fetal nervous system. The brain is smaller, and the basal ganglia (memory, cognition) and cerebellum (balance, gait, coordination, and some cognitive functions) may be affected (Batshaw, 2002, p. 111).

Symptoms: There is a recognizable facial appearance with this disorder and growth retardation. FAS and ARND account for up to 20 percent of all cases of mild mental retardation. Developmental delays in speech and language usually manifest by age 2 (Batshaw, 2002, p. 111).

Prognoses: The outlook for these children is poor. The mothers often lose custody of these children. In one study, 52 percent of FAS children were abused by their mothers. It is necessary to watch the home situation carefully in these cases (Batshaw, 2002, p. 119).

Impact on Family Life and Future Education: These children are usually removed from alcohol-abusing parents. The children need a stable home environment with parents who can give them the time and attention they need. Special schooling, where class sizes are small and the children get lots of one-on-one attention is helpful in many cases.

Diagnosis: PDD (pervasive developmental disorder)

Etiology: These are neurogenetic conditions that affect brain function, and they often co-exist with other diagnoses. The PDD category includes the autism spectrum (autism, Asperger, and PDD not-otherwise-specified [NOS]), plus Rett syndrome and childhood disintegrative disorder (CDD), a very rare condition (Batshaw, 2002, p. 368).

Symptoms: Pervasive developmental disorders all share one primary factor: the inability to communicate appropriately and to respond reciprocally in social situations by age 3, with or without a diagnosis. Language delays are often evident as early as 18 months. Otherwise the individual disorder categories may include rituals; repetitive movements; very limited play skills; restricted emotional response; and in the case of metabolic impairment, degenerating cognitive and physical conditions (Batshaw, 2002, p. 365).

Prognoses: PDD may be the most complex set of disorders in EI, and its incidence is growing as specific patterns of behavior become isolated and identified as new disorders. There are as many specialized approaches to treating these disorders as there are circumstances. Medications, behavioral intervention, and language training are prominent in allowing these children to overcome some of their limitations and to reach higher levels of function.

Impact on Family Life and Future Education: Families will spend much time learning about their child's particular behavioral idiosyncrasies and communication style and how best to discipline when necessary. These children may have stunted emotional growth and delayed communication capabilities (e.g., a 3-year-old may act and speak more like a 1-year-old). There are special education programs specifically for children with autism. The highest-functioning people may be capable of independent living but may always have trouble with relationships because of communication disorders.

Diagnosis: PKU (phenylketonuria)

Etiology: an inborn error of amino acid metabolism caused by an enzyme deficiency (Batshaw, 2002, p. 333).

Symptoms: PKU usually manifests sometime within the first two years of life, signified by degeneration of physical and cognitive skill levels, abnormal gait, behavioral disturbances, and sometimes seizures in untreated individuals.

Prognoses: If a phenylalanine-restricted, low-protein diet is followed, the disease often can be controlled.

Impact on Family Life and Future Education: Children are screened for PKU at birth. If they adopt the proper diet and maintain it, they can lead normal lives. If they do not, they can regress into mental and physical retardation. The most difficult aspect of parenting for these children is to make sure they eat the right foods throughout childhood and adolescence (Batshaw, 2002, p. 334).

Hearing Disorders (Sensorineural and Conductive)

Diagnoses: cochlear dysfunction, cholesteatoma, mastoiditis, voice disorders, resonance disorders, dysarthria, dyspraxia

Etiology: can be genetic, due to such syndromes as CHARGE association (coloboma, heart anomaly, choanal atresia, retardation, genital and ear anomalies), Treacher Collins' syndrome, Waardenburg syndrome, Bardet-Biedl syndrome, Usher syndrome, Down syndrome, trisomies 13 and 18, and cleft palate; if the loss is functional rather than structural, it can be due to complications of infection to the middle or inner ear or throat (Batshaw, 2002, p. 202).

Symptoms: (depend on age) Infants may be unresponsive to sounds; toddlers may not respond appropriately to parents when they speak, may fail to make sounds indicating they want something, may not follow simple commands or understand simple questions, and may not use understandable words.

Prognoses: When hearing loss is not associated with developmental syndromes, the prognosis is good, whether or not the child can hear at all. Cochlear implants are bringing hearing to some children who have never heard sounds before. Hearing aids, American Sign Language, and augmentative communication devices can significantly help many children who have hearing, speech, and language problems.

Impact on Family Life and Future Education: Teaching the child alternate ways of communicating, and learning to use those themselves, are the best ways parents can help. If the child is deaf, special schools exist to serve him or her, or regular classrooms can make accommodations to help the child participate. There is much political activism among the Deaf community, a group of people who have fashioned a culture around their hearing loss.

Musculoskeletal /Neuromuscular Disorders

Diagnosis: Cerebral palsy (CP); juvenile rheumatoid arthritis (JRA); torticollis; brachial plexus injury (Erb's palsy; Klumpke's palsy)

Etiology: CP was once thought to be a disorder of the birth process in which the fetus was deprived of oxygen during delivery. However, for the past 20 years physicians have known that most cases of CP result from premature birth or problems during intrauterine development. Juvenile rheumatoid arthritis is a painful autoimmune disease that inflames the synovium, increases joint fluid, and causes changes in the affected joint. It can involve only one joint or many, or affect the whole body (systemic). Torticollis is a form of dystonia that affects the neck musculature. In Erb's or Klumpke's palsy (brachial plexus injury), the child loses movement in the affected arm. In Erb's palsy, grasp remains intact; however, in Klumpke's palsy, grasp is absent. Ninety percent of brachial plexus injuries resolve on their own within the first six months of life (Batshaw, 2002, p. 66). In the 10 percent of cases that do not resolve, the child is highly limited in the use of one arm and hand. Rehab usually involves accommodation—training the child to use the good arm and hand for activities of daily living (ADL) skills, though assisted grasp with the affected hand may be possible.

Symptoms: In dyskinetic CP, abnormalities in muscle tone involve the whole body, but the involuntary movements are hard to see. Rapid, jerky movements and slow, writhing ones characterize athetoid CP, another type of the disorder. In dystonic CP, there is rigidity in the trunk and neck. Children with ataxic CP display problems with timing and motor movements, difficulty controlling reaching, and an unsteady gait. In mixed or total body CP, a mixture of movement abnormalities is seen. JRA symptoms include fevers, rash, pleural and pericardial effusion, and enlargement of the liver and spleen. JRA is treated with steroidal and non-steroidal anti-inflammatory drugs and topical pain relievers. In torticollis, the neck bends in a painful arch to the side. Torticollis may be present on its own or may be associated with other conditions.

Prognoses: Intelligence is often not affected in CP. If it is not, children have a good outlook for the future as long as they receive coordinated care early, continuing through their school years. JRA is lifelong, and it requires a great deal of accommodation to maintain function. Relieving pain and swelling is paramount, and preventing joint deterioration is most important in the long term. In the worst cases, joint replacement may become necessary. Muscle tone deficits like torticollis are very treatable when they exist on their own. If they are part of a neurological or degenerative disorder, the prognosis is not as good. Therapeutic exercise, adapted play, and positioning help overcome the problem.

Impact on Family Life and Future Education: Children with CP who have normal intelligence should be encouraged to become as independent as possible and to set educational goals for themselves. Overprotection is particularly bad for these children because it projects on them the idea that they are not "good enough" to achieve. Adaptations for mobility and fine-motor skills may be necessary, but these are usually the only tools that such children need to access the same world their peers do. Children with JRA can participate with others to the degree that their energy and pain levels will allow them. Supervised exercise is important to maintaining joint health, and OTs can help these kids get more done with energy conservation techniques. JRA has a very strong psychological component. Stress management and appropriate motivation is very important.

Neural Tube Defects

Diagnoses: spina bifida (meningomyelocele type)

Etiology: This is caused by a single malformation that occurs by 26 days after fertilization of the egg, as the central nervous system is being formed. When the neural groove folds over to become the neural tube, it may not close completely (Batshaw, 2002, p. 469).

Symptoms: In meningomyelocele, a membrane covers the spinal cord, which is deformed, and paralysis results. Hydrocephalis (cerebrospinal fluid in the brain, which leads to enlargement of the head) may accompany meningomyelocele.

Prognoses: Closure of the cord is often possible within days of the birth, but lack of bladder and bowel control may continue to affect children with spina bifida, as well as urinary tract infections, scoliosis, and sensory loss in the legs. These children might require the use of a wheelchair, and most have borderline to average intelligence and often have learning disabilities. They might learn to do physical things, such as wheelchair sports, depending on the extent of their paralysis and the degree of encouragement they get. Eighty-five percent now live into adulthood.

Impact on Family Life and Future Education: Children with meningomyelocele should be given every chance to be as independent as they can and should be encouraged to try new things. They may get depressed or anxious when they cannot "keep up" with peers (Batshaw, 2002, p. 485). They need a lot of care when they are younger, and the family may have to make sacrifices to do this.

Visual Disorders

Diagnoses: Genetic abnormalities: coloboma, retinal defects, cranial nerve palsies, optic atrophy, extreme myopia, retinitis pigmentosa, cataract. Functional/developmental abnormalities: amblyopia, glaucoma, nystagmus, cortical visual impairment, delayed vision maturation, strabismus (Batshaw, 2002, p. 168–177)

Etiology: The genetic eye abnormalities above often are associated with causes that include Aicardi's syndrome, CHARGE association (coloboma, heart anomaly, choanal atresia, retardation, genital and ear anomalies) or Hall-Hittner syndrome (HHS), galactosemia, Lowe syndrome, osteopetrosis, Stickler syndrome, tuberous sclerosis, Tay-Sachs disease, trisomies 13 and 18, and Zellweger syndrome (Batshaw, 2002, p. 168).

Symptoms: Symptoms in these visual disorders range from disrupted visual function to partial vision to blindness.

Prognoses: If the visual problem is functional rather than structural, treatment is usually available. If the problem involves the development of the organ itself, there is often little that can be done medically.

Impact on Family Life and Future Education: Functionally, visual impairments alone do not prevent a child from living a close-to-normal life with environmental and behavioral adaptations, if cognition is unimpaired. However, if the disability is multifaceted, the adapting will be more difficult. Parents might seek resources through the American Foundation for the Blind and through their local Lions clubs, which support the visually impaired.

Other Conditions

Diagnosis: Epilepsy

Etiology: Often seen as a secondary diagnosis in other illnesses, epilepsy is defined as a neurological impairment that is characterized by recurring seizures—a chronic electrical misfiring in the brain.

Symptoms: The seizures that infants may experience from high fevers or acute illnesses are not considered epilepsy. The diagnosis is made according to recurrence and brain wave testing. Seizures may involve involuntary movements of the body, vocalization, loss of consciousness, or suspension of awareness for a short period of time. Seizures are common in many genetically precipitated disabilities.

Prognoses: There are many medications that treat epilepsy. If you observe any type of seizure, have the parent report it to the doctor, and inform the ongoing service coordinator. Prognosis depends on the cause of the seizures. If they are associated with a treatable condition, they may be kept under control. If tumor or brain damage is causing the events, the outlook may not be as good.

Impact on Family Life and Future Education: Epilepsy that is under control does not hamper a normal life. It is a very common disorder. Families may have to adjust the medications for their children and learn what triggers the attacks. These children will not be allowed to drive if their symptoms are not under control.

OF A DIFFERENT MIND

Early diagnosis is key to successful intervention in autism.

By Tisha Nickenig

Children with autism are largely an enigma. What we know about them is far less than what we don't know. Large, distant eyes unmask their fundamental disconnection. Many struggle to interact socially, and some, trapped by their limitations, seek solitude. Their worlds remain secret. And, we, as curious observers, can't find our way in.

Locked outside, we quickly judge what children with autism should look and act like. But when we do this, our understanding of this spectrum disorder gets lost. And so do the children. As a result, many fail to receive a diagnosis until they're 5 or 6. The optimum age, however, should be around 2. The solution is to peer behind autism's facade and sift through the disease's cues. But the telltale hallmarks of autism—failure to understand everyday social interactions, for instance—are often quite subtle, making diagnosis difficult at a young age.

While researchers know a defect exists in the brains of people with autism, they can't pinpoint a specific spot or collection of cells, which makes diagnosis harder, says Catherine Lord, PhD, director of the University of Michigan Autism and Communication Disorders Centers in Ann Arbor, MI. So without a biological marker, clinicians are forced to rely on behavioral observations and family history, which are subjective and always leave room for error.

What clinicians do know is that children with autism have a defect in the neural wiring of the brain. "A fair amount of evidence does exist," says Lord, "that people with autism are processing thoughts in different ways than us, which suggests that their brain grows differently."

People with autism can have sensory disturbances, food allergies, gastrointestinal problems, depression, obsessive compulsiveness, epilepsy, ADHD and extreme anxiety.[2] Most have language delays. Words can come out like a stutter, garbled and sporadic. Frustrated, they may choose more aggressive ways to communicate, such as whoops or deafening shrills.

These symptoms apparently have been known to run in families, manifesting in different forms and severities. "If a child has autism, there's a possibility that a parent has similar social difficulties, such as repetitive or compulsive behaviors," says Lord. In addition, if parents have one autistic child, their chances of having another is about 1 in 20. Studies of identical twins show that if one twin has autism, then the other has a 90-percent chance of being within the spectrum too.[3]

This supports researchers' theories that autism has a genetic component. "We just can't pinpoint it," says Lord. But because the rate among identical twins is less than 100 percent, some researchers also theorize that autism has an environmental trigger.[3]

(continued)

Another mystery—the disorder is four times as likely to occur in boys. Unproven theories abound in research labs, but nothing is determined for sure.

Autism's symptom variability doesn't help solve the riddle. Some people can talk. Others can't. Some have above-normal abilities. Others don't. And some—nearly 25 percent—appear to begin developing normally and then regress.[3]

This heterogeneity makes the disorder difficult to pinpoint. And the sheer number of people with autism complicates matters even further. One in 150 kids aged 10 and younger may be affected by autism or a related disorder, which equals nearly 300,000 children in the United States alone. This makes autism five times more common than Down syndrome and three times as common as juvenile diabetes. If we include adults, according to the Autism Society of America, more than 1 million people are affected by one of the autism spectrum disorders.[2]

Experts have tried to distinguish some of autism's highly variable characteristics by developing subtypes and diagnosing children accordingly. But some question whether these subtypes—known as the autism spectrum disorders—are different forms of the same disorder, or really different altogether.

Along with the variety that exists within the different autistic spectrum disorders, there's also great diversity among them.

Consider the difference between a child with autism and one with Asperger syndrome, an autistic spectrum disorder. The child with Asperger's may have communication issues, but might not have cognitive or clinical delays in language. Nevertheless, he can tend to have problems with the more pragmatic pieces of communication, such as taking turns speaking, says Louanne Rinner, MSED, OTR/L, coordinator of the student-training program at the Kansas University Medical Center, Developmental Disabilities Center in Kansas City. Some children diagnosed with autism, however, can speak, and some children with Asperger's may have difficulty carrying on a conversation with others. So language might not always be the best marker.

Diagnosis is subjective, says Amy Laurent, OTR/L, an occupational therapist affiliated with Communication Crossroads, a private practice in Marlborough, MA. "There have been times a child has been referred to an outside agency for a diagnostic evaluation, because the early intervention team suspects the child may be on the autism spectrum," explains Laurent. "However, when the results of the specialist's evaluation are given, the child often receives a different diagnosis based upon that specialist's interpretation of the child's behavioral presentation." With these diagnostic difficulties in mind, the key to diagnosis is to target the symptoms of each child and try to understand the progression of the disorder.

But that's easier said than done. Many professionals have difficulties distinguishing the whole disorder from its symptoms.[1] If a younger child, for instance, isn't forming friendships in school, he could be displaying autistic characteristics by having no interest in the activities of others. Or he could simply be shy and passive. For this reason, parents are often met with the phrases, "Let's wait and see," or "He'll grow out of it."

(continued)

Even if professionals do suspect symptoms of autism, adds Laurent, they often don't feel comfortable giving the diagnosis. Many times, they don't have sufficient resources or training, and their ability to refer for diagnostic testing may be limited due to the paucity of specialists familiar with diagnosis, explains Laurent. So, to offer families educational services about children with delays, professionals will often refer them to early intervention programs, commonly called birth-to-three programs.

Federal laws require that each state provide early intervention services to infants from birth to 3 years old who have developmental disabilities. Specialists who assess the children in these programs include a wide range of professionals, among them occupational and physical therapists and speech-language pathologists.

While experts agree these specialists are highly motivated and well meaning, they face many obstacles when trying to evaluate children.

"While the programs vary from state to state, many don't emphasize diagnosis because they don't want to label children with the wrong disorder," says Fred Volkmar, MD, professor of child psychiatry at Yale University School of Medicine, New Haven, CT. "But when they avoid diagnosis, they may avoid treatments appropriate for a child on the autism spectrum."

Part of their hesitation comes from the fact that they often work alone in children's homes, and don't have many opportunities to collaborate with experts in other disciplines, says Laurent. "It's very difficult, especially if training opportunities and experienced clinicians aren't prevalent in your community, to go inside a child's home, evaluate them and tell parents you suspect their child has a behavior profile that is consistent with an autism spectrum disorder." It's much easier to concentrate on their difficulties. And that's what many birth-to-three providers do.

"If [the clinician is] an OT, for instance, [she] may primarily evaluate the child from a traditional OT viewpoint," adds Laurent. And this could lead to a clinical diagnosis such as sensory-integration problems, motor delays and/or regulatory difficulties. But these may be just part of the child's difficulties.

That's why programs such as the Autism and Developmental Disabilities Clinic at the Yale Child Study Clinic in New Haven, CT, stress the importance of a specialized multidisciplinary evaluation. Core team members usually include a pediatrician, a psychiatrist, a social worker, a special education teacher, caregivers, occupational and physical therapists, and speech-language pathologists. All contribute to the evaluation process and collaborate to determine a child's behavioral profile.

Emily Rubin, MS, CCC-SLP, a speech-language pathologist who is part of the evaluation team at Yale, for example, evaluates not only whether a child can use language but also whether he can use communicative strategies at the frequency she might expect. She'll also evaluate whether the child can use and respond to nonverbal forms of communication and if he can convey a variety of messages to a partner.

Experts are beginning to do this much earlier than ever before. "We can assess children in the first 3 to 6 months of life by observing how they're beginning to orient to their caregivers through gaze, reciprocal smiling and vocal play," says Rubin. By 6 months,

(continued)

for instance, a typically developing child usually reacts to a caregiver who smiles at him with a reflexive smile. By 9 to 12 months, infants are typically savvy enough to get their parents' attention by crying louder than usual and by sharing nonverbal messages with them, such as pointing or waving.

Lord stresses the importance of involving parents in the evaluation process. If they tell you something isn't quite right and they think their child has a communicative delay, "it's worth taking a second look," she adds. But while it's good to involve parents, it's also vital to evaluate children interacting with people they don't know.

For effective intervention and program planning, professionals need to continue to monitor children's progress, and evaluate their response to treatment, as well as where they started from, explains Lord. This takes time, which many early intervention specialists don't have.

Few specialized clinics and professionals in the country focus their efforts on early diagnosis, says Rubin. Therefore, it's difficult for parents to find professionals who can make an early diagnosis. And when they do, they face costly bills insurance rarely covers and long waiting lists, some as long as 2.5 years.

It's a big problem, but one clinicians and researchers are trying to solve.

A few years ago, Lord and colleagues undertook the somewhat complex task of sifting through the plethora of information about autism. They came up with an observational diagnostic tool to help professionals make an earlier diagnosis: the Autism Diagnostic Observation Schedule. The tool creates situations that attempt to elicit certain behaviors from young children, such as pointing or asking for something. If these behaviors are absent, professionals should be suspicious. Lord's diagnostic tool also includes a parent interview: the Autism Diagnostic Interview-Revised. Physicians or psychologists can ask parents questions about how their child acts in typical situations, which can help them determine a diagnosis of autism.[1]

At the Yale Child Study Center, Dr. Volkmar is working on studies that involve eye tracking in infants and toddlers at risk for autism. In preliminary studies with adolescents and adults, he has used technology to determine where people focus their visual attention while watching a movie. What he and his Yale colleagues observed could change the way we think about people with autism. They looked only at the people who were speaking, and when they did, they never looked above their chin. This finding, along with other patterns that were observed with this technology, could lead to a more objective way of diagnosing infants with the disorder.

It's just a theory right now, a glimpse into what could be. But researchers around the world are testing thousands of these theories through media such as genetic screening, videotaping young children, and functional MRI and EEG testing, which can uncover dysfunctions in the autistic brain. And with every study, they're developing diagnostic tools that will help people assess for the disorder at increasingly younger ages. Their ultimate goal, of course, is to find an early biomarker.

In the meantime, parents try not to get lost in the fog. They concentrate on the facts: every child with autism is different, every case is unique. And they learn that what might be good for one, might not be useful for another.

(continued)

With time, they begin to focus less on the difficulties their child has, and more on who he is and what he can achieve.

References

Azar, B. (1998, November). The development of tools for earlier diagnosis of autism is moving quickly. American Psychological Association. Accessed via http://www.apa.org/monitor/nov98/autism.html

Nash, J. M. (2002, May 2). The secrets of autism: The number of children diagnosed with autism and Asperger's is exploding. Why? *Time.* Accessed via http://www.time.com/time/covers/1101020506/scautism.html

Seven, R. (2001, August 19). Unraveling the deep mysteries of autism: While parents sort the pieces, UW researchers hunt for connections. *Pacific Northwest.* Accessed via http://seattletimes.nwsource.com/pacificnw/2001/0819/cover.html

Resources

Grandin, T. An inside view of autism. Center for the Study of Autism. Accessed via http://www.autism.org/temple/inside.html

The Autism Society of America. What is autism? Accessed via http://www.autismsociety.org/whatisautism.html

Reprinted with permission from ADVANCE for Directors in Rehabilitation, Sept. 1, 2002.

FOOD FOR THOUGHT

- What are some common diagnoses you might expect to see in children referred for early intervention? How important do you feel it is to have the actual diagnosis before you treat?

- The autism syndrome is expanding diagnostically. You will probably see many of these children. Discuss the uncertainties of the diagnosis, as well as its various manifestations. Do you feel you would need more education to handle these cases? Why or why not? How can you use the team to help?

Evaluating a Home Environment 7

NITA'S STORY

Nita was 22 months old. She had been in and out of hospitals over the past 10 months for juvenile arthritis. She had a mop of curls above a moon face caused by corticosteroids. Her hands and feet were also very swollen. She sat on her mother's lap while we reviewed her history and discussed goals: pain management, joint preservation, stress reduction, improving general hand function, and non-restrictive range of motion.

Nita was almost completely dependent in activities of daily living (ADL), so I discussed with her mother how important independence was for Nita's physical development and self-esteem. Nita's mother was holding her five or six hours a day. I suggested that she start putting Nita on the floor in a supported position with a couple of her favorite toys periodically throughout the day. We made a comfortable spot with foam pillows, and she put Nita down. Not a minute passed before Nita started to sob. "I h-u-r-r-r-t, Mommy. Pick me up!" Her mother rushed over to pick her up. I asked her mother to reassure her instead—to tell Nita she was OK and that mommy loved her. Nita's crying escalated to an angry scream. I advised her mother to gradually build up time on the cushions because holding Nita all the time was not good physically or emotionally for either of them.

When I went back two days later, Nita was sitting on the floor holding a small plush animal. She was up to 20 minutes at a time. I suggested we find an old handbag and fill it with small objects for Nita to play with, putting the bag to her right or left, so the child had to turn at the waist. Nita really liked her bag, and her independent play time increased, but progress in other areas was difficult. Her mother said she said she felt "cruel" when she made demands or did not help Nita. Intellectually, she agreed with the therapeutic intentions, but emotionally, she caved in.

Nita was having a flare-up of arthritis the next time I came to see her. Her joints were hot and she was very upset, and so was her mother. I gently asked if anything had happened to raise Nita's stress level, explaining that outside forces could sometimes exacerbate arthritis. Surprised, Mom answered that Nita had heard her parents fighting the night before. Then Nita's mother started to cry and so did Nita. "Can you stop crying and tell Nita that she will be all right and so will the rest of the family?" I asked. She did, and Nita calmed down. Then we talked about asking the doctor if we could use a topical pain lotion on Nita's hand to see if it diminished the pain and swelling a bit.

After Nita's mother got the doctor's approval, I brought a small, hinged, flip-open container that resembled a makeup compact. We put the cream in it so Nita could learn to put on her "make-up" by herself. Her mother felt Nita had not done a good enough job, and finished rubbing it in. I explained that by putting it on as well as she could, Nita was learning a way to help herself. The oral medications were the most important treatment to control the arthritis; the application of the topical cream did not have to be so precise.

Because Nita's mother found participating in her treatment so difficult emotionally, I brought up the idea of center-based treatment for Nita. I reassured Nita's mother that the staff at the center were used to working with children like Nita. I suggested that while Nita was in treatment, her mother should do something she enjoyed. Nita's mother put in an application and a space soon became available. By the time I left, she was relatively comfortable with the idea of Nita going to the center. She made plans to take an art class while Nita was in treatment. Nita would be able to make more progress in her therapy at the center, and the time away would give Nita's mother much respite.

Assessing the Family

Evaluating a family situation is a lot like driving in heavy traffic. You have to focus on what is ahead of you, but you also have to be aware of things around you. You do not refocus on each individual issue as it appears. In the case above, the therapist evaluated the home environment and, though it was generally positive, she identified factors that were impeding the child's progress. In this case, the therapist had a wealth of information on which to base her evaluation. She came to the home knowing the child had a medically diagnosed condition rather than simply symptomatic delays. When she arrived, she saw that the family lived in a well-kept home and that the mother was home with the toddler, who was dressed and ready for therapy. When she observed mother and daughter, the OT discovered that the baby's illness had created some behavioral issues that her mother was emotionally unable to handle. This was causing developmental delays. The mother loved her child very much, and hated to see her cry in pain, but she knew some changes had to be made.

This is a best-case scenario. The family was not wanting for food or employment. The home was clean and safe. The mother would be there to work with her child and to personally discuss issues with the EI therapist. She was obviously eager to help her daughter and was receptive to new suggestions. The therapist could expect a good deal of success here. Unfortunately, in neighborhoods of lower socioeconomic status, the case report above often does not fit the families you will see. You may only be able to talk with a caregiver other than the parents and hope your message gets passed on to them. Even though IDEA encourages a family evaluation, you may have little opportunity to make one when your contact with the parents is minimal. Still, it is possible to learn something about a family's situation by observing the home environment and the caregiver, and it is important for a child's successful treatment that you do so.

Evaluating With the Hierarchy of Needs

Begin your evaluation by observing what fundamental needs the household is working to meet. According to psychologist Abraham Maslow's hierarchy of needs, all human thinking and actions can be categorized according to unmet needs. The first and most basic need is survival. People whose sources of food, water, and shelter are in jeopardy will put securing those things above all else. Next in the hierarchy come safety, love, self-esteem, and self-actualization. The hierarchy of needs can be a useful tool in your evaluation of a home and can help you identify possible challenges to successful treatment (Huitt, 2004).

Is this family ready to participate in treatment?

If the family is primarily focused on surviving, you are not likely to be able to successfully treat a child in that house. The members of the family will be too consumed with securing basic needs to participate effectively in the child's treatment. As you observe the home environment, begin by asking yourself the following questions.

? What is the socioeconomic status of the neighborhood?

? Is the dwelling in serious need of repair?

? Is the child wearing dirty clothes or a dirty diaper?

? If the mother is present, is she well? Is she dressed shabbily or inappropriately?

? How interested is the mother in learning about her child? How does she relate to her child?

? If there is another caregiver, how involved is that person with the child?

? If someone opens the refrigerator, is it nearly empty or full of food offering little to no nutritional value?

? Does the household seem to be in a state of chaos or disorder?

Any one of these things is not sufficient evidence in itself to determine that survival mode is in gear. However, several taken together indicate that the resource level of that family is very low. If you serve in an area of lower socioeconomic standing, you may be saying, "*most* of my families are like that. I have to go in and do therapy anyway. I can't solve all their problems." No, of course you can't. However, if you believe that the child you are seeing is not getting enough to eat or is dangerously neglected, you need to report that to your agency director and perhaps even to child welfare authorities, depending on your state laws.

Part of the problem in deciding how to assess or handle a situation in which you suspect the family is struggling for basic necessities lies in not having enough information. Often, you will not be able to meet the parents during daytime sessions because both of them are working. In some cases, there will simply be nobody home when you show up. A certain number of no-shows can lead to a family's automatic discharge, depending on the agency.

Your agency administrator or case manager will be able to tell you what services are being provided to a particular family if you are concerned about their welfare. If you decide, after talking about the case, that there are resources you need to refer the family to, do so, but do not allow yourself to become preoccupied with solving all of a family's problems. Your goal is to help your clients help themselves. One very important aspect of best practice is not to be overcome either by sympathy or cynicism. Empathy is the appropriate response: it is a practice skill and part of the therapeutic use of self.

Is this family fearful?

Personal safety is one step up Maslow's ladder from survival (Huitt, 2004). In most environments you will work in, safety needs are psychological in nature, but in some cases physical safety is also an issue. Threats to individual family members or to the family unit can include weapons or other life-threatening items left in places where children can reach them, unsafe stairs or windows, domestic violence (physical and emotional), involvement with drug dealing or street gangs, drug or alcohol abuse, impending bankruptcy, unexpected job loss for any reason, arrest or impending imprisonment, involvement in a lawsuit, or dealing with the stress of a catastrophic or terminal illness or injury.

When people are afraid they behave in certain ways. Children may hide from you or, conversely, try to "attack" you by behaving in a threatening manner. Frightened children may also show a flat affect or seem disconnected from those around them. Adults who are afraid are wary or nervous. They may not want to let you in, may try to cancel the session abruptly, or they may hurry through it in a distracted manner. They will answer questions in only a sentence or two.

If what you are seeing and hearing tells you intuitively that this is a fearful household, check it out. Ask if there is some concern the parent or caregiver would like to share. If they say yes, make them aware that though you cannot promise to keep it confidential, depending on the nature of the concern, you can help them get the help they need. If you feel unsafe in a home, leave immediately. If you suspect, from observation or interaction with caregivers or others, that the child in the home is not physically safe, this *must* become your first priority.

Call your agency and report your observations. Sometimes, a talk with the agency administrator will disclose information that you were unaware of—the situation has been reported and child welfare evaluators have been there, or other members of the team are working on these issues. If you still feel the need to ensure the child's safety, discuss what should be done, and make sure you follow up on it.

Safety issues can be transitory. That is, individuals living in a home may feel safe at some times and not others. For example, a battered wife may feel safe when her husband is not drinking. If the threat is financial or medical, you may not know of it unless the family chooses to divulge it. Underlying any of these types of threats is a constant sense of fear that is hard to dispel. If you sense that the people you are talking to are nervous, preoccupied, or putting up some kind of front for you, safety issues (real or imagined) may well be involved.

Does the relationship between mother or caregiver and child seem to work?

Love, simply put, is kindly contact or attention, and is necessary for good health throughout a person's life. Observing the interaction between mother or caregiver and child can give you information about whether a child's need for love is being adequately met. Do they smile at one another? Do they touch? Do they seem to communicate with each other effectively?

We all need other people. This is why human beings do so many things in groups. The family is the most important group to which we belong, and it needs a sense of cohesiveness to be strong. When parents are under stress they may fail to give their children the care and attention they need, and family cohesion begins to break down. The most important part of your job is modeling for parents or caregivers how to give loving, effective attention to their children.

Does the toddler like to show off his or her skills, either verbally or physically?

Self-esteem is the image we have of ourselves at any given moment. We consciously or unconsciously judge our own worth by that image and by how it compares with the values we hold. Love is a prerequisite for self-esteem and we learn to love ourselves through being loved by others. Lack of love perpetuates itself and deprives its victims of the ability to love others.

Self-esteem also rests on perceived personal competence reinforced by a loved and respected other. In young children, this sense of competence is an important marker of self-esteem. Is the child afraid to try new things? Can he or she show different kinds of feelings? Does the child do the things he or she is capable of doing independently or does the child ask the mother for help?

It is important that caregivers not talk down to a child or help him or her over obstacles that can be managed alone, even if it takes a little longer. If a child is overly dependent and self-esteem seems to be suffering, it is important to teach the family to foster the child's competence. Although it takes patience, each little victory is a building block for the next one and contributes to a child's positive self-image.

Infants and young children can have their self-esteem damaged by circumstances that are beyond their control. They may believe they are responsible for problems between their parents or other negative situations in the household. Parents need to make sure that children understand that adult issues and problems are not their fault. The emotional connection that feeds self-esteem is consensual validation—the acceptance and support of another who cares. Each person we love, each place we feel safe, and each role we play to our satisfaction becomes part of us.

Self-actualization, the highest level of Maslow's needs scale (Huitt, 2004), occurs when the individual can determine his own path, even if it is different from that of others. Self-esteem coupled with validated adult skills and maturation eventually leads to self-actualization. It creates positive energy and enables a person to become who they want to be and live the life they want to live.

Working With the Family or Caregiver

Your role as an advocate for and advisor to your client families can be a difficult one. Chances are you are not a clinically trained counselor, but many times, the parents of a severely disabled child are hurting as badly as their child. They are often weary from 24-hour-a-day vigilance over the health and safety of their children with disabilities. There may be trouble between the parents. They need to learn coping mechanisms—to care for themselves as well as their children. They may feel like children themselves and slip into a state of depression and dependency. The more you can bring out the courage inside them, the stronger they will feel and act. Sometimes it is necessary to remind them what grown ups are capable of dealing with. To do this effectively, you must acknowledge their feelings with empathy and objectivity. You cannot see clearly to help anyone if your emotions are leading you.

To begin this process, you first need to listen to their grief or anger and accept them; understand the situation from their points of view. This is difficult to do when you have to put your own value system aside to understand theirs. What they want for their child may not be what you think is most important, but you need to meet them where they are: that is what empathy is. Often this is enough to begin a relationship. Some therapeutic relationships grow quickly and easily because the two people involved share similar perspectives on life. When they do not, it is the therapist's job to find the key that unlocks the door to the client's thought processes and the attitudes and beliefs that support them.

You must come to understand your client's attitudes and beliefs so that you can work effectively together in carrying out a plan of treatment for the child. Parents need to be taught to help their child when you are not there. The hour or two per week that the child spends with you may not be enough to achieve therapeutic goals in a timely manner. Caregivers need to be competent and comfortable carrying on the games, exercises, and tasks that enhance the child's life and help them to reach the goals the family set.

Interviewing Caregivers

Parents are usually very concerned with their child's growth and development, whether or not they are able to be present for therapy. If there is a parent present, you have a great opportunity to start helping members of the family participate in their child's treatment and to learn as much as you can about the family with whom you will be working. Parents will usually be able to provide you with invaluable information about the child's health, behavior, and role within the family. Talk informally with the parents or caregiver about the child's situation. Do not begin by asking specific questions about the child's delays. Instead, make your questions open-ended, so that the parent has a chance to talk about the big picture and what he or she believes contributes to the child's issues. "What do you consider your child's problem to be?" is a good question to open with.

Some parents will be very specific in their answers. They may have done a lot of their own research and may be able to describe in great detail what their child is having trouble with. Others will be less informed, but their impressions can give you valuable clinical information as well. Once you have discussed the parents' overall impressions of the child's status, use the child's IFSP, which the parent helped create, and the doctor's diagnosis (if you have it) to frame questions that are specific to functional development. You want to find out what the parent is most concerned about and why. Be prepared to answer the parents' questions about their child to the best of your ability.

Parents are likely to consider you an expert, so never dismiss a question. If you do not know the answer, offer to find the information or give a resource where the answer might be found. Parents are usually highly interested in receiving a child's prognosis, but because EI therapists often have no medical diagnosis and only a sheet of evaluation findings and treatment goals to work with, it is sometimes hard to determine one. You may need to use your observational and interviewing skills to dig a little deeper into a child's case before you are able to comment on prognosis. Sensitivity is essential when discussing a child's problems and likely prognosis with the parents. It is important not to give a parent false hope, but it is also important not to crush illusions on which parents lean for support in the early months of caring for a baby with severe physical or developmental delays.

Uncovering the Family Dynamics

Ask questions that will give you information about the relationship between parent and child. "Are you having any trouble handling your child?" is a good opening question. Discussing the parent's impressions of the child's behavior gives you essential information about the parent/child relationship as well as the opportunity to begin teaching the parents the coping skills they may need.

All people want to control their environment so that it meets their needs. Adults have the tools and power to do this for themselves; children are literally at their parents' mercy. Children recognize they are not capable of complete independence, and though they want and need their parents to set boundaries, they will often challenge those limits. Children with disabilities are no different, but parents often treat them as though they are. Parents of children with disabilities are sometimes afraid to discipline their children because they feel they "have gone through so much already," however, external discipline now leads to self-discipline later. As pruning stops the tree from sapping its own strength by growing wild, so rules and responsibilities give children strength and competence.

Parents of children with disabilities often make the mistake of setting low expectations for their child. Low expectations guarantee limited achievement. When a child behaves in an unruly way while you are there, suggest and model ways to set appropriate boundaries. Parents will learn from you how to change their child's behavior by changing their responses to it. Remind them to talk in "I" sentences: (e.g., "I feel bad when you ignore me and jump on the furniture.") and to criticize the action rather than the person (e.g., "Throwing your toy at your sister was wrong. Please go apologize.").

Toilet training is a common issue in children with disabilities. Often children are still in diapers even after their elimination has become regular and they are aware of when they need to go. Toilet training is a self-mastery issue. Once a child becomes old enough to be aware of having to use the toilet, he or she wants to avoid soiling the diaper. The child wants to control his or her own body. It is very important to encourage this, by cheerfully taking the child to the toilet at regular intervals, and saying that soon she will be able to wear "big-kid" pants. Talk about toilet training if you feel you need to. Parents may need to be educated about it.

One of the most common problems EI therapists encounter in homes is dependency. In order to learn to do things, children must have access to opportunities. Some families unwittingly close off the child's opportunities to meet developmental milestones. Parents may not want the child to pick up tiny objects because he or she might put them in his or her mouth. They will not let toddlers have finger foods for fear of choking. Some will not encourage their child to learn to ask for things, responding instead to pointed fingers. Scissors are dangerous, crayons are off limits, and paints are too messy to use. Of course it is wise to be protective, but parents need to create opportunities for their children to get the practice they need in gross- and fine-motor activities and in speech.

Whatever the issues in the parent-child relationship are, modeling will be one of your most effective tools in teaching the parents to care for their child. What the family sees you do, they can imitate. No amount of instruction can take the place of modeling. It is often necessary to assign "homework," as the therapist did in the case study at the beginning of the chapter, because children need to practice their skills daily in order to develop. This type of homework is also a psychosocial aid that helps bring the family together, and it should be fun. Simply helping parents play with their children is a good first step.

Therapists are "outsiders," and because they are trained to help a child realize his or her maximum potential despite disability, they can sometimes elicit better responses than parents. Nevertheless, gaining a child's trust takes time. You cannot rush into a house for the first visit and expect to handle a baby or toddler. If the environment is chaotic or the child is ill, re-schedule the appointment. You need to let the child come to you. To accomplish that, you will have to interest the child in something you have or are doing.

Never coerce a child to do anything. All relationships are two-way, and they take time and patience to build. Modeling this is one of the most important lessons you can teach. The more a parent treats a child with a disability like any other child, the more likely that child is to perform at his or her maximum potential.

Obtaining a Child's Medical Information

Your treatment plan in medically involved cases is determined by the child's medical status. Therapy should not disrupt the medical routine, but should aid and complement any medical care the child is already receiving. Part C of IDEA makes it clear that providers are to be given the medical information necessary to evaluate and effectively treat infants and toddlers. Often medical diagnoses are missing from the IFSPs, since their inclusion is not required. Physicians are often reluctant to make definitive diagnoses in the 0–3 population, so in some cases no diagnosis has been made yet. Instead, an IFSP might list only the child's current abilities plus functional problems that need to be remediated or accommodated.

In the case of major illness, the lack of diagnosis can be a significant hindrance, but most cases seen in early intervention are not critical. The children are referred not because of a diagnosed critical illness but simply because the parents are concerned about on-time development. "Doctors may say, 'well, we're seeing this symptom and that symptom, so we need to take a look at the situation,'" Barbara Chandler, IDEA advocate and a long-time OT educator now based at James Madison University in Virginia, when asked about the diagnosis issue. "It's not cut and dried." Sometimes, doctors are simply unwilling to divulge a child's medical information, but this is rare. It was once possible to pick up a phone and call the referring physician to discuss the case, but current HIPAA rules forbid that without the *written* consent of both parents *and* doctor. Do not hesitate to ask the parents for their signature and permission. The doctors will usually comply.

Dealing With a Language Barrier

The caregiver or parent is the person primarily responsible for meeting the child's needs, and it is important that you be able to communicate effectively with them. If you do not speak the same language, the family may request that your agency send in another therapist who can speak the family's native language. If this is not possible, it is your duty to ask your agency for an interpreter. Unfortunately, getting an interpreter is not always easy, and you may have to rearrange your treatment schedule to accommodate a third person in the process. Sometimes family members who speak both languages can be helpful in these situations.

Assessing Developmental Delays

Although parents' impressions of and concerns about a child's development determine the goals of EI therapy in any given case, developmental evaluations can also form an important part of determining a treatment plan. When administering any kind of developmental evaluation, therapists need to use their professional evaluation skills to carefully interpret the results. In order to accurately assess whether a child has a delay in a particular area, a therapist will need to recognize a skill (or lack thereof) in more than one activity. If you rely exclusively on one activity to demonstrate a child's skills, you may falsely identify a developmental delay where none exists. For example, one child could not complete a pegboard activity, and so the evaluating OT marked him as delayed in fine-motor skills. When the treating therapist arrived, she found that the parents had to be very careful with pill bottles, because their son had opened one, taken out the pills, and put them, one at a time, into slots in his toys! The child had been unable to use the pegboard simply because he had never played with one before, not because he lacked fine-motor skills.

To effectively determine a delay in a given area, you need to begin testing skills that are below the age level of that child, and then work up to skills that are beyond it. When you evaluate in this way, you will be able to place the child somewhere on that continuum. Because you are working with very young children, you need to evaluate them for very small gains in skill level over a period of time to accurately identify a delay.

If you are the evaluating therapist, but someone else will be treating the child, write your findings in very general terms that will allow the treating therapist to choose his or her own tools to treat and even to refine the evaluation. Be aware that the tools you have and use in treatment may be different from what others use, and avoid recommending specialized treatment approaches.

FOOD FOR THOUGHT

- How would you determine a child's prognosis in the absence of a diagnosed medical condition?

- Do you believe most parents love their children? If so, why might they be neglectful or incompetent caregivers?

- What is "modeling," and why is it so important in early intervention?

Concluding Therapy, Keeping Current

8

MIKE'S STORY

Mike was 13 months old when he was referred to EI. He was not walking or talking and he had poor fine motor skills—no pincer grasp or in-hand coordination. He had been placed in daycare at three months when his mother returned to her executive position in a large company. Mike's daycare class had 7 children near 12 months old. He was the only one not walking or even trying to walk. He was the fastest crawler I had ever seen though. Even up ramps or stairs, he out-crawled the fastest walker.

His behavior was appropriate in reading group and during meals. He waited his turn at snacks, was attentive and seemed to understand the stories—clapping or smiling with the others. But Mike did not play well with other children. He would snatch toys away and refuse to give them up, instead holding them tightly to his chest. He was empathetic to the other children, however. He would crawl over to a crying child and pat him or her while making soothing, soft, "lu-lu-lu-lu" sounds.

I met with his mother and explained to her that I thought Mike had not mastered hand control because he had little opportunity to practice it. Daycare centers with many young children do not usually focus on fine motor tasks, because they require closely supervised time with small objects. I gave Mike's mother some silk bags with a few small items in each. I showed her how to present one object at a time, taking it in pincer grasp with my own thumb and index finger from one hand to the other, then offering it to Mike. He tentatively reached for and took a bright red stone from me with his index finger and thumb, and grinned from ear to ear. I held open the bag. "Please put it back," I said, and he did that too. His mom was amazed. She admitted that she had never offered him small objects at home because her older son, who was very jealous of the baby, made it difficult for her to focus exclusively on Mike. "Can you work with Mike in the high chair?" I asked. "Can your husband play with the older child for 10 minutes when you do?" She agreed to try, and it worked.

I asked the daycare to let me play with Mike and a few other children in a corner of the classroom. After several sessions, I had the children handing objects to each other and back again, saying "please" and "thank you." Mike was learning to share and began to say "peez" and "anks." He also began to copy the other children who were pulling themselves up to stand to walk. One day he pulled himself up and tentatively took a few steps toward the snack table, where he grabbed his chair. Everyone clapped, even the other children. Mike's grin lit up the room!

After six weeks of work with Mike, I scheduled another session with his mother. She was pleased with Mike's progress and pleased with herself. Mike had begun to feed himself with a spoon and was taking more steps. She also noted that since her husband had begun playing with their older son while she worked with Mike, the two boys were getting along better. "You taught me therapy techniques and gave me confidence. I can see Mike responding and improving every day. Do you think he needs more OT?" she asked. "No, I don't. I think you have everything under control. A skilled mother is more important than the best OT!" With a tear in her eye and a relieved smile, she hugged me.

When and How to Discharge Patients

Traditionally, under IDEA Part C, all government-funded EI services ended by the time children were 3 1/2 years old. With the 2004 reauthorization of the law, however, states may now connect their early intervention and preschool programs to keep children in necessary services until they are 5, without interruption. States are not required to do this, but it is something for which EI providers might want to advocate with their states' lead agencies.

A child may be discharged from EI regardless of age if he or she meets IFSP goals in a particular discipline. With disabilities like torticollis, for instance, this is fairly clear-cut. (Can he move his head in all planes? Fully visually scan his environment? Crawl on all fours? Use both hands?) But with more comprehensive mental and or physical involvement like Down syndrome, autistic disorder, or cerebral palsy, children are seldom discharged from therapy. They move on to preschool and then to school-based programs, because pervasive problems require continued therapy. As these children age, their IFSPs are changed to reflect their developmental needs. Discharge from EI may also occur if the child misses a number of sessions without notice. Such children may be referred to center-based programs instead of home-based ones.

Transitioning to Preschool

Transitional processes are built into the EI system, and most parents are made aware of those processes before it is time to transition. Nevertheless, parents may be apprehensive about their child entering preschool. It is uncharted territory. They may fear that "the system" will label children according to growth levels in a way that is very unforgiving of individual circumstances and differences. Preschool teachers, who have learned to appreciate these differences between children more than most EI therapists have, are often able to reassure parents that they understand children exist in a state of becoming; they are not set in stone.

Sometimes parental anxiety about a child being unfairly labeled is aggravated by therapists' tendencies to communicate prescriptively. Sometimes therapists are quick to make judgmental statements about what they have observed in a child because they think in terms of cases, not people. This is a holdover from the clinical setting, but it should not be happening there either. Early interventionists should learn to think more like teachers in this respect, because that is what they are.

It is important that EI discharge summaries include general recommendations, but specific recommendations should be avoided because preschool therapy differs from EI in several significant ways. Preschool programs are educational rather than developmental, and they focus on school-based issues. In general, preschool therapy is not as family-oriented as EI, although therapists may still involve the family when appropriate. Additionally, EI is a better-funded program than preschool, and children may have fewer services or fewer sessions in preschool therapy.

Ethical Issues of Discharge

EI cases are funded for one year at a time, so a child who needs occupational therapy twice a week has 104 sessions open. To the agencies and therapists, this is a calculable cash flow and creates a tendency to use up all available hours. The rationale is that there is always more one can do to enhance the skills of a young child. This same tendency has become established in special education.

It is not only bad practice, but fraudulent use of public money, to keep a child in therapy who has either met or cannot ever meet functional goals, with or without adaptation. Functional goals are occupational goals (e.g., holding a cup, putting on shoes, eating with a utensil). Too often therapists whittle down functional goals into skill subsets, and use mastery of the subsets as goals. This can become an endless string of practice activities instead of therapy with a meaningful endpoint. Your agency should discourage this practice, and should not discourage you from discharging a child whose parents are now able to give the child the help he or she needs to meet realistic goals. If your employer wants you to keep children in treatment after they no longer need it, remind the employer that it is your clinical, professional opinion that the child no longer needs OT, and document the fact in your notes.

Whether you will encounter issues over discharging patients depends on the agency for which you work. One therapist at a county health department in New York State (where EI falls under health care rather than education), found that the county encouraged discharge from a service when the child had met IFSP goals and was functioning at his maximum potential, no matter how low. The philosophy was to help the child become part of his family unit by ensuring the family knew how to take care of him.

For-profit agencies tend to want to keep cases open. One school-based provider agency told a therapist that it did not even know the procedure for discharge. "When I found out through the school how to discharge and had the agreement of parents and school staff to do so, I discharged five MR/DD teens," the therapist said. "The agency had a fit! 'If you didn't want to work with them, we have other therapists who do!' I realized that the agency was counting on the $5,000+ a year those kids brought in." Since these services are funded by taxpayers, best practice in discharge requires a real commitment to honesty on the part of the provider. This does not mean that children should not get the care they need; it means that clinicians must be highly skilled in assessing when children are ready to conclude therapy and in preparing the parents to take charge of a child's care.

If parents insist on keeping their children in therapy beyond what you believe is needed, the agency can assign the child to another therapist; but in most cases, when parents feel confident in their ability to continue working with their children, they will agree that home visits are no longer needed. Parents, not endless therapy, are the key to a child's continuing progress.

Keeping Up With the Field: Should You Be Certified in EI?

Early intervention is not dominated by any one discipline. Though occupational and physical therapists and speech-language pathologists are mentioned in the law as qualified providers, in at least 35 states, paraprofessionals may be used. In most states, certification or credentialing in EI is still voluntary, but as EI becomes more well-defined, standards will change, and therapists will have to demonstrate their competencies in EI. Most states began to develop certification and credentialing standards for EI 10 years ago, mostly at the paraprofessional level. Professional therapists in the three major rehab disciplines continue to practice according to the dictates of their licensure regulations, under the rules of the agencies that employ them. Twenty-three states now have, or are in the process of, designing and implementing credentialing for early intervention personnel (University of Connecticut, A.J. Pappanikou Center, 2003). Because skill levels are so widely divergent, there is some question as to what will best prepare an individual for EI practice. Many preschool or school-based therapists try their hands at early intervention at some point, but a school setting does not provide an opportunity to work with severely disabled infants. The best kind of preparation for EI is from a clinical setting, in a hospital NICU or pediatric unit. Unfortunately, most early intervention therapists do not have that background.

Some states have already begun to institute mandatory certification to ensure knowledge of child development and child services among EI professionals and paraprofessionals. Many offer free training, either at schools within the state or through state agencies. Check with the lead agency in your state to find out what you need to do to become credentialed as an early interventionist. Massachusetts has a comprehensive professional development tool in EI, which includes a self-appraisal checklist covering specific competencies and categories. Disregarding the few areas which apply specifically to Massachusetts state law, compare your experience and knowledge base to the competencies in Figure 8.1, and you will get an excellent picture of how close you are to being able to do best practice in early intervention. (You can access the full, interactive self-evaluation tool online at www.eitrainingcenter.org. Click "certification," to open the tool.)

The Massachusetts initiative is a good example of the type of programs more states are likely to institute as the push for credentialing in EI gains momentum. Most EI certification or training programs are offered through administration-education cooperatives, in which lead agencies interpret their needs according to IDEA, and colleges create curricula to meet those needs. Certifying states usually offer these courses for free, with flexible scheduling to help students work around their other obligations.

The certification movement has been led by national teaching organizations, which began pushing for standards in 1994, when the Division for Early Childhood (DEC) of the Council for Exceptional Children issued a position paper, "Personnel Standards for Early Education and Early Intervention." Over the past 10 years, two other organizations, the National Association for the Education of Young Children (NAEYC) and the Association of Teacher Educators (ATE) have reaffirmed their positions in favor of professional credentialing in EI. They believe credentialing standards should be outcome-based, not course-based (avoiding creating another profession), and that graduate level training should be part of a career ladder in early intervention (DEC, 1994).

As more states require certification in early intervention through university-based programs, there will be a need for more clinical training sites in EI. EI has a wealth of information to offer students simply because it is so varied in casework and so rich in person-to-person relationships. Home-based EI rounds could greatly enhance level-one clinicals in pediatrics. Using EI sites for level-2 fieldwork should be carefully planned. Students cannot work alone here because there is no one nearby to ask for clinical information and support. Students should never be given their own caseloads in early intervention as part of a level-2 affiliation. It is essential that students visit homes and work in tandem with experienced practitioners. Under the close guidance and supervision of a mentor, students will find the EI setting highly educational and interesting.

Competency Area 1: Infant and Toddler Development

Competency Indicator	Entry 1 (Knowledge Sources)	Entry 2 (Professionalism)	Entry 3 (Depth of Practice)	Entry 4 (Breadth of Practice)
1.1 Demonstrate knowledge of theories of infant and toddler development, including content, sequences, range and variability within developmental domains.	✓		✓	
1.2 Demonstrate knowledge of etiology, characteristics of common developmental disabilities and risk factors as well as their effect on early development and child-caregiver interactions.		✓		✓
1.3 Demonstrate knowledge of the impact of prematurity on development.	✓			✓
1.4 Demonstrate knowledge of the impact of environmental, cultural, family, biological and health/medical influences on child growth and development, as well as access to information sources and techniques to address the impact.	✓		✓	
1.5 Summarize the implications of recent brain research on child growth, development and learning opportunities.	✓		✓	
1.6 Describe a child's play behaviors across developmental domains and identify intervention strategies..	✓		✓	
1.7 Incorporate caregiver/child interactions in outcomes and strategies.	✓		✓	

Competency Area 2: Evaluation and Assessment

Competency Indicator	Entry 1 (Knowledge Sources)	Entry 2 (Professionalism)	Entry 3 (Depth of Practice)	Entry 4 (Breadth of Practice)
2.1 Collect, interpret and report information from available records.			✓	
2.2 Demonstrate knowledge of the functions of various evaluation and assessment procedures and instruments (screening, standardized evaluation, criterion-referenced assessment, ecological assessment and assessments to help families determine their priorities, resources and concerns).	✓		✓	
2.3 Conduct family interview and incorporate information into other team assessment data.			✓	
2.4 Initiate pre-assessment planning with the family, including facilitating the participation of the family in the assessment at the level desired by the family.			✓	

(continued)

Figure 8.1   Self–Evaluation Tool for EI Competencies

Competency Area 2: Evaluation and Assessment *(continued)*

Competency Indicator	Entry 1 (Knowledge Sources)	Entry 2 (Professionalism)	Entry 3 (Depth of Practice)	Entry 4 (Breadth of Practice)
2.5 Demonstrates knowledge of state eligibility criteria, ability to conduct eligibility evaluation, and ability to interpret information to family and team.	✓		✓	
2.6 Individualize and adapt assessment procedures to meet the special needs of the child, the culture of the family and the variety of contexts of the child's daily life (home, community settings, child care).	✓		✓	
2.7 Administer a criterion referenced assessment instrument to determine child progress and demonstrate the ability to discuss the results by communicating effectively with family members.			✓	
2.8 Demonstrate skills in alternative methods of assessment including: informant interview, behavior rating scales, parent-child interaction and observation of daily routines and play environments.	✓		✓	
2.9 Collaborate with the family to identify current level of functioning, strengths and needs of the infant/toddler.	✓		✓	
2.10 Demonstrate cultural responsivity throughout the evaluation and assessment process.	✓			✓
2.11 Conduct an environmental assessment of an infant/toddler child care or community setting to determine how an infant/toddler can be supported in that environment.			✓	

Competency Area 3: Family Centered Services and Supports

Competency Indicator	Entry 1 (Knowledge Sources)	Entry 2 (Professionalism)	Entry 3 (Depth of Practice)	Entry 4 (Breadth of Practice)
3.1 Demonstrate understanding of the roles, responsibilities and relationships of families in caring for and educating young children with disabilities, including recognition of strengths and resources that families contribute to the child's development.	✓		✓	
3.2 Demonstrate knowledge of family-centered principles and the ability to apply family-centered principles to services and supports while working in collaboration with families.	✓		✓	

(continued)

Figure 8.1   Self–Evaluation Tool for EI Competencies *(Continued)*

Competency Area 3: Family Centered Services and Supports (continued)

Competency Indicator	Entry 1 (Knowledge Sources)	Entry 2 (Professionalism)	Entry 3 (Depth of Practice)	Entry 4 (Breadth of Practice)
3.3 Demonstrate knowledge of family systems theory, interactions, and how a disability effects family functioning.	✓		✓	
3.4 Demonstrate understanding and respect of the diversity and individuality of family functioning, including influences of culture and ethnicity.	✓		✓	
3.5 Demonstrate leadership in advocating for families to meet concerns and priorities for their child and family.			✓	
3.6 Share complete and unbiased information with families to enhance their ability to weigh the pros and cons of services, supports and techniques.			✓	
3.7 Provide a flexible menu of participation and support opportunities for families regarding identification, implementation and evaluation of child and family outcomes and strategies.			✓	
3.8 Demonstrate the ability to evaluate family centered communication skills through self-assessment.		✓		

Competency Area 4: Individualized Family Service Plan (IFSP)

Competency Indicator	Entry 1 (Knowledge Sources)	Entry 2 (Professionalism)	Entry 3 (Depth of Practice)	Entry 4 (Breadth of Practice)
4.1 Explain the IFSP process to promote a family's comfort level and participation in the process.			✓	
4.2 Facilitate the IFSP meeting and record decisions made regarding outcomes, strategies and services.	✓		✓	
4.3 Demonstrate skills and knowledge to generate functional outcomes and strategies with the team, including the parents.	✓		✓	
4.4 Develop IFSPs that meet IDEA regulations and DPH Operational Standards.	✓		✓	
4.5 Prepare the family and other team members for the review of the IFSP.			✓	

Figure 8.1   Self–Evaluation Tool for EI Competencies *(Continued)*

Competency Indicator	Entry 1 (Knowledge Sources)	Entry 2 (Professionalism)	Entry 3 (Depth of Practice)	Entry 4 (Breadth of Practice)
5.1 Use effective communication skills and productive problem-solving or mediation strategies as a team member with a variety of audiences.			✓	
5.2 Demonstrate knowledge of specialty service providers, public/private community providers, their rules and requirements to network and advocate in order to increase options for children and families.	✓		✓	
5.3 Demonstrate skills to create natural learning opportunities for young children and a sense of belonging for families.	✓		✓	
5.4 Implement plans to promote smooth transitions for children from EI to Early Childhood Special Education or other community programs.	✓		✓	
5.5 Coordinate and maintain regular communication with medical and health care professionals for individual children.			✓	
5.6 Identify and assist a family to access other financial resources for their child (Medicaid, SSI, CHIP).			✓	
5.7 Monitor and coordinate the delivery of early intervention services on the IFSP.			✓	
5.8 Coordinate and schedule evaluations, IFSP meetings and reviews to meet timelines.			✓	
5.9 Demonstrate knowledge of local, regional, state and federal agencies that focus on the social, financial, health, developmental and other needs of infants/toddlers and their families.			✓	
5.10 Advocate for resources needed by families and enhance the family's capacity for self-advocacy.			✓	

Figure 8.1   Self-Evaluation Tool for EI Competencies *(Continued)*

Competency Area 6: Intervention Strategies

Competency Indicator	Entry 1 (Knowledge Sources)	Entry 2 (Professionalism)	Entry 3 (Depth of Practice)	Entry 4 (Breadth of Practice)
6.1 Create and adapt learning environments that enhance infant/toddler learning opportunities and positive behaviors in natural settings.	✓		✓	
6.2 Use activity-based intervention to integrate individual needs of infants/toddlers within activities and routines.			✓	
6.3 Develop strategies for intervention based on individual strengths and needs of the family.			✓	
6.4 Plan for and implements home visits designed to produce positive outcomes for children and families.			✓	
6.5 Use a daily routine format to embed individual outcomes and strategies for a child throughout the day/week.	✓		✓	
6.6 Combine developmentally appropriate practice with functional intervention strategies to individualize across developmental domains.	✓		✓	
6.7 Demonstrate the ability to lift, carry, position and facilitate mobility and function for a child with disabilities.				✓
6.8 Plan for health, nutrition and feeding needs of specific infants and toddlers.	✓			✓
6.9 Support an infant's or toddler's learning and sensory needs.	✓		✓	
6.10 Teach others to implement specific strategies to adapt routines/equipment that promote the acquisition of skills and active participation in age appropriate activities.			✓	
6.11 Design and implement individual activities using adaptive and assistive technology to facilitate a child's participation and autonomy.	✓			✓

Figure 8.1   Self–Evaluation Tool for EI Competencies *(Continued)*

Competency Area 7: Team Collaboration

Competency Indicator	Entry 1 (Knowledge Sources)	Entry 2 (Professionalism)	Entry 3 (Depth of Practice)	Entry 4 (Breadth of Practice)
7.1 Demonstrate knowledge of the role, functions and composition of different team models.	✓		✓	
7.2 Facilitate team or IFSP meetings through agendas, preparing families and delineating responsibilities.			✓	
7.3 Serve as a resource and consultant to the family and team members regarding information and methods specific to her/his own discipline to promote the optimal development of the infant/toddler.	✓		✓	
7.4 Collaborate and consult with other agencies and community programs to provide needed services without duplication, gaps or delays.			✓	
7.5 Demonstrates ability to utilize negotiation and conflict management techniques.	✓		✓	
7.6 Demonstrates understanding of the different roles and competence of different disciplines.	✓		✓	
7.7 Consistently evaluate with team members the effectiveness of services being delivered to adapt to any changes in infant/toddler or family.			✓	

Competency Area 8: Policies and Procedures

Competency Indicator	Entry 1 (Knowledge Sources)	Entry 2 (Professionalism)	Entry 3 (Depth of Practice)	Entry 4 (Breadth of Practice)
8.1 Demonstrate a basic knowledge of relevant federal and state legislation, regulations and policies (including IDEA, FERPA, MASS EI Standards, and vendor policies) that impact services and supports to children and families.	✓		✓	
8.2 Demonstrate knowledge of due process and procedural safeguards and the ability to communicate the purpose and content of each to all families served.	✓		✓	

Figure 8.1   Self–Evaluation Tool for EI Competencies *(Continued)*

Competency Area 9: Professionalism

Competency Indicator	Entry 1 (Knowledge Sources)	Entry 2 (Professionalism)	Entry 3 (Depth of Practice)	Entry 4 (Breadth of Practice)
9.1 Participate in opportunities for continued training and education.		✓		
9.2 Periodically use self-evaluation for the purpose of targeting goals and specifying steps to ensure ongoing personal professional growth.		✓		
9.3 Demonstrate flexibility in response to diversity and change.		✓		
9.4 Demonstrate professional work habits including dependability, time management, independence and responsibility.		✓		
9.5 Demonstrate knowledge of current research concerning efficacy of early intervention.		✓		
9.6 Demonstrate appreciation for diverse perspectives, needs and characteristics of individuals.		✓		
9.7 Demonstrate use of current Early Care and Education, Early Intervention, or Early Childhood Special Education, or pediatric research literature to solve problems and/or modify practice.		✓		
9.8 Contributes to the body of knowledge in the field by participation in professional organizations, studies, sharing of data, writing and/or presenting information.		✓		

Early Intervention Specialist Competencies, Massachusetts Department of Public Health, reprinted with permission.

Figure 8.1   Self–Evaluation Tool for EI Competencies

Current Research in EI

Any child development study may contribute to the body of knowledge that applies to early intervention, but there is a lot of direct research going on in the field itself. As of May 2005, the Resources to Practice Division of the U.S. Department of Education's Office of Special Education Programs (OSEP) was supporting more than 1,000 projects in educational research through discretionary grants and contracts around the country, funded through IDEA. About 470 of them are in the 0–2 or 0–3 category, and all 50 states are involved. You can access the project database at http://www.cec.sped.org/osep/database/showAllage.html to find out exactly where studies are underway, what is under scrutiny, and when projects will be completed. Some of the research projects now underway involve virtually every aspect of disability seen in early intervention, including blindness/low vision, deafness/hearing loss, speech and language deficits, communication deficits, autism, mental retardation, serious emotional disturbance, developmental delay, specific and general learning disabilities, attention-deficit hyperactivity disorder, orthopedic disabilities, multiple disabilities, cross-categorical issues, traumatic brain injury, and professional development in early intervention.

Research and EI Outcomes

Current research is helping therapists to achieve family-focused practice in EI. In the mid 1990s, The Early Childhood Institute on Measuring Growth and Development set out to research the success of family outcomes in early intervention. Researchers from the universities of Minnesota, Kansas, and Oregon wanted to produce a system to continuously measure the skills and needs of children with disabilities from birth to age 8. The system would incorporate not only growth and development indicators for children but resources for families and teachers as well, offering information on how to modify children's environments to create the best opportunities for growth and learning. Interviews with the parents of children with disabilities revealed what they wanted most from early intervention, including:

- understanding the law as it pertains to the IFSP/IEP process
- understanding basic child development and being able to assess how their child is developing
- understanding their child's disability and knowing how to access supports within the community related to that disability
- being able to identify their own needs as a family, including those related to culture, linguistics, or disability-specific issues
- being made aware of their resources as soon as a need is identified, and to have information on how to access those services
- receiving the services they have identified as being necessary in a timely manner
- perceiving themselves as equal and integral members of the team
- having confidence in their abilities to make choices about services for their children
- being self-advocates
- understanding the differences between IFSP and IEP procedures and the resulting implications for service provision
- feeling that other members of the team respect their beliefs and values

Out of this investigation, the Child Research Institute created the "Family Outcomes in a Growth and Development Model." It identified four potential family outcomes that fit its comprehensive assessment model focused on the child's growth and development. EI professionals might use some of the following criteria to measure their effectiveness in family-based intervention:

1. Families should have a basic understanding of child development and be able to identify the needs of their child, including those related to cultural, linguistic or disability-specific issues. You can assess this by observing the level of family participation in meetings over time. You can also use self-evaluations and family satisfaction surveys to get a picture of what is happening.

2. Teach your families to refer back to the outcomes identified on the IFSP to assess their child's developmental progress. Let them participate in the monitoring process using the same basic tools you use, and then assess their success through self-evaluations and participation in intervention design.

3. Under this model, it is critical that there is consistency between professionals and families in implementing interventions. Team members together determine the impact of the child on daily family routine, and what adaptations the family is willing to make to that routine in order to implement the interventions.

4. Let your families know that you respect their beliefs and values. The families will then see themselves as equal and integral members of the team.

Having included family participation in all phases of the process, the final family outcome measures overall family satisfaction with the outcome of that process.

The Move Toward Evidence-Based Practice

While the explosion of research in the field is undeniably positive for early intervention, there is a simmering debate over the value of different kinds of research in EI practice.

The mantra "evidence-based practice" was ringing in the ears of health care professionals and educators even as the latest reauthorization of IDEA became law on December 3, 2004. The reauthorization of IDEA says that services are to be based on scientifically proven methods to the extent practicable. Congress is using the term "evidence-based practice" to try to establish standardization in therapy practice and to ensure efficacy in therapeutic methods.

The potential problem with the move to evidence-based practice is that evidence-based means different things to different people. To nurses and doctors, it refers to applying clinically researched treatments, considered to be "of choice" in the industry, to particular medical conditions. To educators, evidence-based may involve using a long-established but not necessarily scientifically proven protocol—using phonics to teach reading, for example.

The current political climate is moving to apply medical research standards to all clinical applications, including behavioral ones. That is, lawmakers want to see every interventional tool tested for efficacy. They do not want to be told that it works. They want to know how or why it works, and they want you to be able to point them toward the studies that prove it does.

EI employers may begin applying higher standards of practice to the therapists they employ to ensure compliance with the law. As the law now reads, such evidence should be used "to the extent practicable." No one knows just how tools would be qualified if there were such a requirement in a future version of IDEA, or who would do the judging. It is not even clear at this point if such qualifications would apply to early intervention. It would be a good idea, however, to start cataloguing some research on the tools you use most often in therapy. Do not look for randomized, double-blind studies. You are not likely to find them. Just gather a small foundation of applied research that you can use to back up your tools if you have to. The American Occupational Therapy Association is now collecting such information. You can access its Web site at www.aota.org.

Early intervention is a challenging setting and one that is worth committing yourself to. You can make more of a difference here than in almost any other setting you might choose, for this is where it all begins, not only for the infant or toddler, but for mom and dad, brother and sister. Achieve best practice in EI, and you will be a skilled practitioner, mentor, and educator.

FOOD FOR THOUGHT

- What are the ethical issues that arise in discharging children from early intervention?
- What kind of evidence do you think is most necessary for research-based OT practice in this field? How would you acquire it?

References

Amen, D. G. (2001). *Healing ADD: The breakthrough program that allows you to see and heal the 6 types of ADD.* New York: Putnam.

Barnett, W. S. (2002, September). *The battle over Head Start: What the research shows.* Paper presented at a congressional Science and Public Policy briefing, Washington, DC.

Batshaw, M. (2002). *Children with disabilities* (5th ed.). Baltimore: Brookes.

Brazelton, T. B., & Nugent, J. K. (1995). *The neonatal behavioral assessment scale.* Cambridge University, United Kingdom: Mac Keith Press.

Civitas Initiative, Zero to Three, & Brio Corporation. (2000). *What grownups understand about child development: A national benchmark survey.* Retrieved August 10, 2005 from http://www.zerotothree.org/parent_poll.html

Commons, M. L., & Miller, P. M. (1998, February). *Emotional learning in infants: A cross-cultural examination.* Paper presented at the American Association for the Advancement of Science, Philadelphia, PA.

Dickerns, W. T., & Flynn, J. R. (2001). Heritability estimates versus large environmental effects: The IQ paradox resolved. *Psychological Review, 108*(2), 346–369.

Division for Early Childhood (DEC). (1994). *Position statement on personnel standards for early education and early intervention.* Retrieved August 10, 2005 from http://www.dec-sped.org/pdf/positionpapers/Position%20Personnel%20Standards.pdf

Early Childhood Outcomes Center. (2005). Family and child outcomes for early intervention and early childhood special education. Retrieved August 10, 2005 from http://www.fpg.unc.edu/~eco/pdfs/eco_outcomes_4-13-05.pdf

Fassler, D. G., & Dumas, L. S. (1997). *Help me, I'm sad: Recognizing, treating, and preventing childhood and adolescent depression.* New York: Viking Penguin.

Goleman, D. (1995). *Emotional intelligence: Why it can matter more than IQ.* New York: Bantam.

Hawes, J. M. (1999). *The great IQ wars: Struggles behind the ideas that supported project Head Start.* Retrieved August 10, 2005 from www.connectforkids.org/articles/struggle_behind_head_start

Herrnstein, R. J., & Murray, C. (1994). *The bell curve: Intelligence and class structure in American life.* New York: Free Press.

Heyrman, C. L. (2000). *Religion, women, and the family in early America.* Retrieved August 10, 2005 from http://www.nhc.rtp.nc.us:8080/tserve/eighteen/ekeyinfo/erelwom.htm

Huitt, W. (2004). *Maslow's hierarchy of needs.* Retrieved August 10, 2005 from http://chiron.valdosta.edu/whuitt/col/regsys/maslow.html

Hwang, Y. G. (1997-98). Let's strike out: Self-esteem rhetoric in special education. *National Forum of Special Education Journal, 6*(1-2), 23–26.

Individuals with Disabilities Education Act of 1997, Public Law 105–17 (IDEA Reauthorized), U.S. Statutes at Large (1997).

Individuals with Disabilities Education Improvement Act of 2004, Public Law 108–446, U.S. Statutes at Large 118 (2004): 2647.

Jones, H. W., Jr., & Schrader, C. (1987). The process of human fertilization. *Fertility and Sterility, 48*(2), 189–192.

Kleiman, M. A. R., (2003). *Environment, IQ and Head Start*. Retrieved August 10, 2005 from http://www.samefacts.com/archives/000133.html

Kotulak, R. (1996). *Inside the brain: Revolutionary discoveries of how the mind works*. Kansas City, MO: Andrews McMeel Publishing.

Maldonado, M. (2003). *Culural issues during pregnancy*. Retrieved August 10, 2005, from www.kaimh.org/slides/cultural

Orr, S. T., Miller, C. A., James, S. A., & Babones, S. (2000). Unintended pregnancy and preterm birth. *Paediatric and Perinatal Epidemiology, 14*, 309–313.

Peterson-DeGoff, M. (2005). *Developmental care: Overstimulation and your premature baby*. Retrieved August 10, 2005 from http://www.prematurity.org/overstimulation.html

Shattock, P. (1995). The use of gluten and casein free diets with people with autism. Retrieved August 10, 2005 from http://osiris.sunderland.ac.uk/autism/dietinfo.html

Skeel, H. M., Updegraff, R. , Wellman, B., & Williams, H. M. (1938). A study of environmental stimulation: An orphanage preschool project. *University of Iowa Studies in Child Welfare, 15*(4), 1–191.

Strydom, J.& du Plessis, S. (2003). The role of genetics in IQ and intelligence. Retrieved August 10, 2005 from http://iq-test.learninginfo.org/iq03.htm

Tucker-Ladd, C. E. (2000). *Psychological self-help*. Retrieved August 10, 2005 from http://mental-help.net/psyhelp/

University of Connecticut, A.J. Pappanikou Center. (2003). *Study I data report: The national landscape of early intervention in personnel preparation standards under part C of the Individuals with Disabilities Education Act (IDEA)*. Retrieved August 10, 2005 from www.uconnucedd.org/Publications/files/PPDataPartCweb.pdf

U.S. Department of Health and Human Services. (1999). *Mental health: A report of the Surgeon General*. Retrieved August 10, 2005 from http://www.surgeongeneral.gov/library/mentalhealth/home.html

Ventura S. J., Abma J. C., Mosher W. D., & Henshaw S. (2003). Revised pregnancy rates, 1990–97, and new rates for 1998–99: United States. *National Vital Statistics Report, 52*(7), 1–14.

Wilcox, A. J., Weinberg, C. R., O'Connor, J. F., Baird, D. D., Schlatterer, J. P., Canfield, R. E., et al. (1988). Incidence of early loss of pregnancy. *New England Journal of Medicine, 319*(4), 189–194.

Yale Child Study Center. (2003). *History of the child study center*. Retrieved August 10, 2005 from http://www.med.yale.edu/chldstdy/history.html

Zero to Three. (n.d.). *Developmental milestones: How I grow in your care*. Retrieved August10, 2005 from http://www.zerotothree.org/dev_miles.html

Zero to Three. (2000). What Grown-Ups Understand About Child Development: A National Benchmark Survey. Retrieved August 10, 2005 from http://www.zerotothree.org/parent_poll.html